Teenagers and AIDS in America

Edited by
J. Stango

Nova Science Publishers, Inc.

Art Director: Christopher Concannon
Graphics: Elenor Kallberg and Maria Ester Hawrys
Manuscript Coordinator: Roseann Pena
Book Production: Tammy Sauter, and Michelle Lalo
Circulation: Irene Kwartiroff and Annette Hellinger

Library of Congress Cataloging-in-Publication Data

Teenagers and AIDS in America / J. Stango, editor.
p. cm.
Includes bibliographical references and index.
ISBN 1-56072-178-2
1. AIDS (Disease) in adolescence--United States.
I. Stango, J.
RJ387.A25T44 1994 94-6979
362.1'969792'00835--dc20 CIP

6080 Jericho Turnpike, Suite 207
Commack, New York 11725
Tele. 516-499-3103 Fax 516-499-3146
E Mail Novasci1@aol.com

Printed in the United States of America

TEENAGERS AND AIDS IN AMERICA

CONTENTS

CHAPTER I

MILLIONS OF AMERICAN YOUTH ARE AT RISK FOR HIV INFECTION †

HIV is transmitted through sexual contact (vaginal, oral, and anal), contaminated needles or syringes, infected blood or blood products, transplanted tissue or organs from an infected donor, and from mother to fetus.[1]

The number of adolescents currently infected with HIV is unknown. Authorities have reported relatively few cases of AIDS among teens. However, substantial evidence indicates that thousands of adolescents are already infected with HIV and millions of youth are at risk of infection.[2]

The extent to which the HIV epidemic has spread in any population is estimated by a variety of methods, including AIDS case surveillance, HIV seroprevalence studies, and surveys of HIV risk factors such as sexual and drug use behaviors.[3] This chapter discusses the findings and limitations of each of these methodologies as used with adolescents.

A. THE EPIDEMIOLOGY OF AIDS AMONG ADOLESCENTS -- NEARLY 9,000 YOUNG ADULTS ALREADY DIAGNOSED WITH AIDS

AIDS case surveillance data provide a readily available method of tracking the spread of HIV. These data, collected by the Centers for Disease Control (CDC), indicate gradual changes in the spread of the HIV epidemic and the emergence of populations that are at risk of infection.[4] It is important to note, however, that AIDS case surveillance data only track the end stage of HIV infection, thereby significantly underestimating its progression.[5] Changes in the spread of HIV will not be reflected by patterns of AIDS cases for years.[6]

For example, the number of teens diagnosed with AIDS is relatively small. However, nearly one-fifth of all U.S. AIDS cases have been reported in persons ages 20-29. The best estimates

† Excerpted from CRS Report 102-1074

available indicate that the mean incubation period between HIV infection and clinical diagnosis of AIDS is eight to ten years.[(a)] Therefore, it is unlikely that persons infected during their teenage years would be diagnosed with AIDS as teens. As noted by the National Research Council:

> Even with the assumption of a median incubation period of eight years, fewer than one-half of persons infected with HIV at age 13 would be expected to develop AIDS during their teenage years, and even fewer of those infected in the late teens would develop AIDS before age 20. Those persons who are diagnosed with AIDS during their teens will be drawn mainly from the group of persons whose incubation periods were markedly shorter than the median and who were infected during their early teens.[7]

Other limitations of using AIDS case data to estimate the extent of the HIV epidemic are related to problems with reporting the data. AIDS cases may be under-reported by as much as 20% in a number of states, including those with a high prevalence of HIV infection.[8]

Further, CDC reports AIDS case data for adolescents in broad age groups (13-19 and 20-24) rather than by specific age at diagnosis. These age groupings are somewhat arbitrary and confusing. By the end of 1991, 789 cases of AIDS had been diagnosed in youth ages 13-19. However, by adding cases among youth ages 20-21, the total more than doubles to 2,552, and by adding young adults ages 22-24, the total number of AIDS cases more than triples again to 8,949.[(b)] Since many services are available to adolescents through age 18 or 21, many experts advocate for presenting AIDS case data by specific age at diagnosis or by narrow age groups.[9]

(a) The incubation period may depend on the route of transmission and the age of the individual infected. Natural history studies of hemophiliacs infected with HIV suggest that adolescents and children remain asymptomatic longer than adults. [Miller, H.G., et al. (eds.) 1990. op cit.]

(b) For the purposes of this report, recognizing the limitations described above, AIDS case data will be presented according to the broad age groups currently reported by CDC.

In addition, without requesting a special data run by CDC, it is impossible to determine by gender, both the mode of transmission and the race/ethnicity of AIDS cases within the broad age groups. These data are particularly important because as will be illustrated in this chapter, the mode of transmission varies significantly between females and males and by race and ethnicity.

Finally, the definition of AIDS has changed several times since it was first identified more than a decade ago to more accurately reflect the opportunistic diseases that indicate advanced HIV disease in women, children and adults. CDC has recently proposed expanding the definition of AIDS for adolescents and adults to include people with severe HIV disease. This change would nearly double the number of people in the U.S. with AIDS by including an additional 160,000 persons.[10]

AIDS Cases Among Youth Rising Quickly

As shown in Table 1 and Figure 1, the number of AIDS cases in young adults has increased dramatically in recent years, with more than half of all cases in persons ages 13-24 having been reported in the last 36 months of the decade-long epidemic.

Table 1: Cumulative AIDS Cases Reported Each Year In Persons Ages 13-24, By Age Group[(c)]

Year	13-19	20-24	13-24
1981	1	6	7
1982	3	35	38
1983	11	125	136
1984	35	303	338
1985	71	645	716
1986	130	1,263	1,393
1987	211	2,204	2,415
1988	333	3,622	3,955
1989	461	5,063	5,524
1990	628	6,694	7,322
1991	789	8,160	8,949

(c) Special data request prepared by Reporting and Analysis Section, Surveillance Branch, Centers for Disease Control. August 1, 1991, and January 13, 1992. Numbers are reported from January through December for each year.

Figure 1: AIDS Cases Among Adolescents and Young Adults Ages 13-24, By Age Group, Reported Through 1991[(d)]

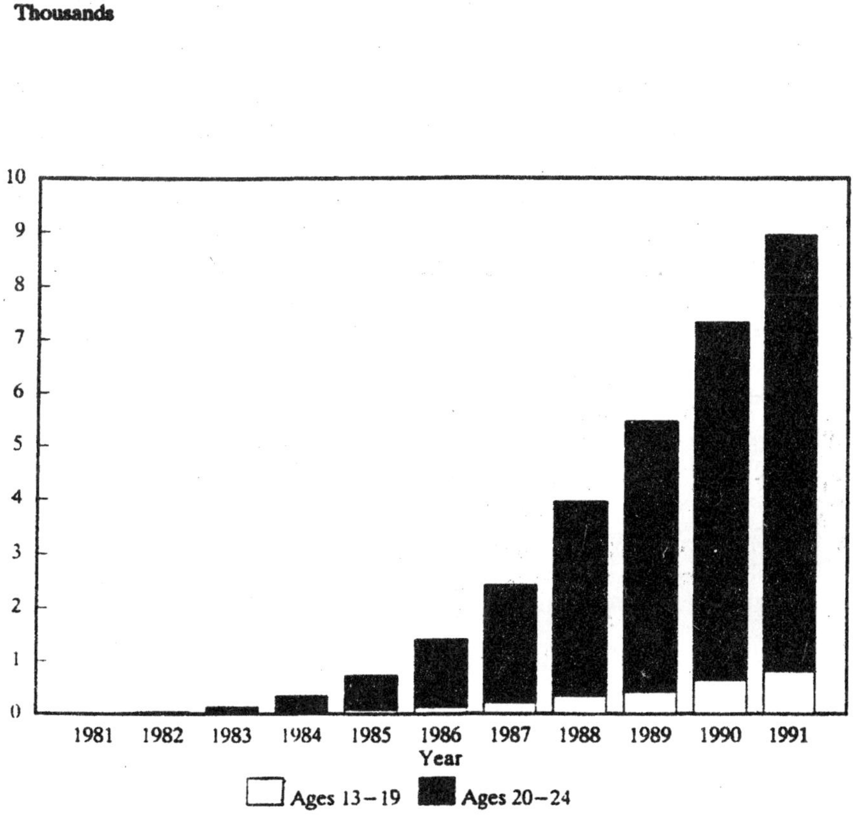

(d) Special data request prepared by Reporting and Analysis Section, Surveillance Branch, Centers for Disease Control. August 1, 1991, and January 13, 1992. Numbers are reported from January through December for each year.

Heterosexual Transmission More Common Among Youth, Smaller Proportion of AIDS Cases in Youth Related to Injecting Drug Use

The epidemiology of AIDS cases among teens and young adults (ages 13-24) differs from that of older adults in several important ways. Adolescents and young adults are more likely than adults to have acquired the virus through heterosexual transmission, or as a result of exposure to contaminated blood and blood products, and are less likely to have been infected as a result of homosexual activity or injecting drug use.

As shown in Table 2, the mode of transmission varies significantly by gender. Transmission through heterosexual contact accounts for 45% of AIDS cases among teenage females, compared with 2% of AIDS cases in males ages 13-19. It should also be noted that a large proportion of AIDS cases among young teens is related to hemophilia in males or blood transfusions. By mid- and late adolescence, however, the mode of transmission shifts dramatically to sexual transmission (both heterosexual or homosexual).[11]

Table 2: AIDS Cases Among Adolescents and Adults, By Gender and Exposure Category, Reported Through 1991[e]

Exposure Category	Ages 13-19		Ages 20-24		Ages 25 & Older	
	Number	Percent	Number	Percent	Number	Percent
MALE -						
Men who have sex with men	197	(34.1)	4,462	(66.0)	113,703	(65.2)
Injecting drug use	44	(7.6)	856	(12.7)	34,148	(19.6)
Men who have sex with men and inject drugs	33	(5.7)	731	(10.8)	12,371	(7.1)
Hemophilia/coagulation disorder	238	(41.2)	203	(3.0)	1,230	**
Heterosexual contact	12	(2.0)	200	(3.0)	4,475	(2.6)
Receipt of blood transfusion, blood components or tissue	27	(4.7)	64	**	2,588	(1.5)
Other/undetermined	26	(4.5)	249	(3.7)	5,839	(3.3)
Male Subtotal	**577**		**6,765**		**174,354**	
FEMALE -						
Injecting drug use	57	(26.9)	550	(39.4)	10,098	(51.5)
Hemophilia/coagulation disorder	4	(1.9)	4	**	34	**
Heterosexual contact	96	(45.3)	657	(47.1)	6,496	(33.1)
Receipt of blood transfusion, blood components or tissue	26	(12.3)	53	(3.8)	1,589	(8.1)
Other/undetermined	29	(13.7)	131	(9.4)	1,401	(7.1)
Female Subtotal	**212**		**1,395**		**19,618**	

** = less than one percent

(e) CDC. January 1992. op cit.; Special data run January 13, 1992. Division of HIV/AIDS, Center for Infectious Diseases, Centers for Disease Control. Totals may not add to 100% due to rounding.

Females and Minorities Represent Greater Proportion of Cases of AIDS in Youth

Among individuals with AIDS, younger adults and teens are more likely than older adults to be female and members of a racial or ethnic minority group. While the majority of U.S. AIDS cases are reported among men, women now account for more than 10% of all U.S. cases among adolescents and adults (ages 13 and older). In fact, during 1991, the number of AIDS cases among adolescent and adult women increased by 37%, compared with 27% among men.[12]

Comparing the ratio of AIDS cases between men and women provides further evidence of the important role that heterosexual transmission of HIV plays among teens and young adults.[13] Among AIDS cases diagnosed in persons ages 25 or older, nine men are diagnosed for each diagnosis among women. In cases among persons ages 20-24, the ratio of males to females is less than five to one, and in teens it drops to less than three cases among males for each case reported among females.

Racial and ethnic minority populations are disproportionately represented among AIDS cases at all age levels. This is especially true among teens and younger adults. As shown in Table 3, compared with AIDS cases among adults over age 24, African-American, Hispanic, and other racial and ethnic minority youth account for a greater proportion of AIDS cases among persons under age 25. While African Americans represent 15.2% of the U.S. population ages 13-19, they represent 37% of all AIDS cases reported in that age group. Similarly, Hispanics represent 11.7% of the teens, but 19% of AIDS cases reported among persons ages 13-19.[f]

(f) Based on 1990 Census data, 80.2% of the U.S. population ages 13-19 is white, 15.2% is African-American, 3.5% is Asian/Pacific Islander, and 1.1% is American Indian/Native American. Teens with Hispanic origin represent 11.7% of the U.S. population ages 13-19, however, Hispanic persons may be of any race. Therefore, the percentages noted here reflect overlapping groups. Special data run, U.S. Department of Commerce, Bureau of the Census, Population Division. March 2, 1992.

Table 3: AIDS Cases Among Adolescents and Adults, By Gender and Race/Ethnicity, Reported Through 1991[g]

	Ages 13-19		Ages 20-24		Ages 25 and older	
Gender	Number	Percent	Number	Percent	Number	Percent
Male	577	(73%)	6,765	(83%)	174,354	(90%)
Female	212	(27%)	1,395	(17%)	19,618	(10%)
Total	**789**		**8,160**		**193,972**	
Race/Ethnicity						
White, not Hispanic	332	(42%)	3,703	(45%)	105,611	(55%)
Black, not Hispanic	292	(37%)	2,757	(34%)	55,144	(28%)
Hispanic	151	(19%)	1,612	(20%)	31,261	(16%)
Asian/Pacific Islander	8	(1%)	48	(1%)	1,202	**
American Indian/Alaska Native	6	(1%)	18	**	290	**
Unknown	0	na	22	**	464	**

** = less than 1%

(g) CDC. January 1991. op cit.; Special data run January 13, 1992. Division of HIV/AIDS, Center for Infectious Diseases, Centers for Disease Control. Totals may not add to 100% due to rounding.

AIDS Cases Among Teens and Young Adults Reported in 49 States and Nearly 100 Large Metropolitan Areas

AIDS case data also indicate that the epidemic has spread quickly from the early epicenters that included New York, California, and Florida. By the end of 1991, 44 states and the District of Columbia had reported AIDS among teens, and 49 states and the District of Columbia had reported AIDS cases among young adults age 20-24. (See Table 4)

Table 4: AIDS Cases in Persons Ages 13-24, By State and Age Group, Reported Through 1991[(h)]

State of Residence	Age Group 13-19	Age Group 20-24	Age Group 13-24
Alabama	11	83	94
Alaska	1	10	11
Arizona	7	97	104
Arkansas	7	50	57
California	80	1116	1196
Colorado	11	64	75
Connecticut	7	95	102
Delaware	1	19	20
District of Columbia	6	146	152
Florida	86	874	960
Georgia	27	279	306
Hawaii	2	29	31
Idaho	0	5	5
Illinois	31	257	288
Indiana	10	65	75
Iowa	1	12	13
Kansas	5	34	39
Kentucky	8	43	51
Louisiana	17	171	188
Maine	2	18	20
Maryland	16	191	207
Massachusetts	16	171	187
Michigan	15	104	119
Minnesota	2	47	49
Mississippi	8	58	66
Missouri	24	150	174
Montana	2	5	7
Nebraska	0	9	9
Nevada	0	41	41
New Hampshire	3	14	17
New Jersey	46	429	475
New Mexico	3	16	19
New York	103	1272	1375
North Carolina	18	118	136
North Dakota	0	0	0
Ohio	19	135	154
Oklahoma	5	44	49
Oregon	2	49	51
Pennsylvania	37	246	283
Rhode Island	1	18	19
South Carolina	11	71	82
South Dakota	0	2	2
Tennessee	8	83	91
Texas	57	760	817
Utah	3	21	24
Vermont	2	3	5
Virginia	8	128	136
Washington	9	98	107
West Virginia	1	11	12
Wisconsin	6	35	41
Wyoming	0	4	4
Subtotal	**745**	**7800**	**8545**
Guam	0	0	0
Pacific Islands	0	0	0
Puerto Rico	44	355	399
Virgin Islands	0	5	5
Total U.S.	**789**	**8160**	**8949**

(h) Special data request prepared by Reporting and Analysis Section, Surveillance Branch, Centers for Disease Control. January 13, 1992. Note: CDC surveillance data list the District of Columbia as a state of residence.

Table 5 illustrates the number of AIDS cases among teens and adults under age 25 reported in large metropolitan areas. These data show that by the end of 1991, AIDS cases had been reported among youth in nearly 100 large metropolitan areas. These data also indicate that while AIDS cases continue to be reported primarily in large metropolitan areas, by the end of 1991 nearly one-third of AIDS cases among youth ages 13-19 were outside of metropolitan areas with populations of 500,000 or more.[14]

Table 5: AIDS Cases in Persons Ages 13-24 in Metropolitan Areas Having Populations of 500,000 or More, By Age Group, Reported Through 1991[(i)]

Metropolitan Area of Residence	Age Group 13-19	20-24	13-24
Akron, OH	1	9	10
Albany/ Schenectady, NY	2	19	21
Allentown, PA	0	8	8
Anaheim, CA	4	62	66
Atlanta, GA	16	197	213
Austin, TX	3	58	61
Bakersfield, CA	1	13	14
Baltimore, MD	10	103	113
Baton Rouge, LA	2	12	14
Bergen-Passaic, NJ	9	61	70
Brimingham, AL	1	29	30
Boston, MA	10	126	136
Bridgeport, CT	0	28	28
Buffalo, NY	2	13	15
Charlestown, SC	2	10	12
Charlotte, NC	1	16	17
Chicago, IL	24	214	238
Cincinnati, OH	4	15	19
Cleveland, OH	7	36	43
Columbus, OH	2	29	31
Dallas, TX	7	154	161
Dayton, OH	1	13	14
Denver, CO	3	44	47
Detroit, MI	9	69	78
El Paso, TX	0	13	13
Fort Lauderdale, FL	11	134	145
Fort Worth, TX	2	51	53
Fresno, CA	0	12	12
Gary/ Hammond, IN	2	4	6
Grand Rapids, MI	0	9	9
Greensboro, NC	3	16	19
Greenvile, SC	2	8	10

Metropolitan Area of Residence	Age Group 13-19	20-24	13-24
Harrisburg, PA	4	9	13
Hartford, CT	2	26	28
Honolulu, HI	0	20	20
Houston, TX	20	276	296
Indianapolis, IN	1	30	31
Jacksonville, FL	6	47	53
Jersey City, NJ	5	65	70
Kansas City, KS	13	84	97
Knoxville, TN	0	7	7
Lake County, IL	0	3	3
Las Vegas, NV	0	28	28
Little Rock, AR	0	13	13
Los Angeles, CA	31	421	452
Louisville, KY	2	20	22
Memphis, TN	3	37	40
Miami, FL	17	216	233
Middlesex, NJ	2	32	34
Milwaukee, WI	2	24	26
Minneapolis/ St. Paul, MN	0	40	40
Monmouth/ Ocean City, NJ	3	22	25
Nashville, TN	0	19	19
Nassau/ Suffolk, NY	10	55	65
New Bedford, MA	0	13	13
New Haven, CT	5	35	40
New Orleans, LA	5	103	108
New York, NY	77	1078	1155
Newark, NJ	18	177	195
Norfolk, VA	3	44	47
Oakland, CA	5	74	79
Oklahoma, OK	3	25	28
Omaha, NE	1	3	4
Orlando, FL	1	56	57

(i) Special data request prepared by Reporting and Analysis Section, Surveillance Branch, Centers for Disease Control. January 13, 1992.

Metropolitan Area of Residence	----- Age Group ---- 13-19	20-24	13-24
Oxnard/ Ventura, CA	1	11	12
Philadelphia, PA	24	203	227
Phoenix, AZ	6	63	69
Pittsburg, PA	2	23	25
Portland, OR	2	34	36
Providence, RI	1	16	17
Raleigh/ Durham, NC	1	31	32
Richmond, VA	1	26	27
Riverside-San Bernadino, CA	7	74	81
Rochester, NY	3	26	29
Sacramento, CA	3	27	30
Saint Louis, MO	7	66	73
Salt Lake City, UT	1	19	20
San Antonio, TX	10	60	70
San Diego, CA	7	102	109
San Francisco, CA	10	211	221
San Jose, CA	4	33	37
San Juan, PR	22	192	214
Scranton, PA	2	8	10
Seattle, WA	5	54	59
Springfield, MA	5	12	17
Syracuse, NY	3	11	14
Tacoma, WA	0	21	21
Tampa- Saint Petersburg, FL	14	105	119
Toledo, OH	0	12	12
Tuscon, AZ	1	23	24
Tulsa, OK	0	11	11
Washington, DC	13	258	271
West Palm Beach, FL	15	108	123
Wilmington, DE	1	10	11
Worcester, MA	1	13	14
Metropolitan Area Subtotal	552	6550	7102
All Other Areas	237	1610	1847
Total	789	8160	8949

B. SEROPREVALENCE STUDIES INDICATE RAPID SPREAD OF HIV AMONG ADOLESCENTS

The CDC estimates that approximately one million Americans are currently infected with HIV and that at least 40,000 new HIV infections occur each year among adults and adolescents.[15] As noted previously, while AIDS case data provide a readily available source of data about the HIV epidemic, they severely underestimate its spread. Probability samples of the prevalence of HIV infection among individuals drawn from well defined populations would provide a more accurate assessment of the extent of the epidemic.[16] With few exceptions, however, HIV seroprevalence studies are drawn from samples of convenience which do not include adolescents.[17]

Seroprevalence studies based on nonprobability samples that have included adolescents and young adults have found a wide range of HIV infection. For example, among the nearly 950 youth ages 15-19 who used an STD clinic in Baltimore during a four-month period in 1987, 2.2% (or about one in 50) were infected with HIV. Among patients ages 15-24 who were served by a Bronx hospital during a nine-month period in 1988, 3.6% of males and 2.5% of females were infected with HIV.[18] In New York City, one in 170 teenage women (under age 20) who delivered live births between November 30, 1987 and March 31, 1990 was infected.[19] By contrast, among students served by 17 U.S. college health units between 1988 and 1989, 0.2% (or one in 500) was infected with HIV.[20]

To date there are no national epidemiologic studies of HIV infection among adolescents. The lack of population-based data makes it impossible to accurately estimate the prevalence of HIV infection among adolescents. The largest samples for national seroprevalence studies involving adolescents have come from applicants for U.S. military service and Job Corps[(j)] entrants.[21] (See Table 6 for summary.)

(j) Job Corps is a Federally-funded educational and training program to help economically disadvantaged youth (ages 14-21) complete their education and learn skills that will help them obtain employment.

Table 6: Comparison of HIV Infection Rates Among Young Military Applicants and Job Corps Entrants[k]

Description	Military Applicants	Job Corps
Dates of Data Collection	October 1988-March 1989	October 1987-February 1990
Number of Youth Tested	1,141,557	137,209
Race and Ethnicity of Study Population		
White	837,544	41,409
African American	215,869	75,036
Hispanic	55,630	14,024
Other	32,514	6,440
Age of Study Population	17-19 years	16-21 years
Percent with HIV infection among study population	0.03%	0.36%
Percent with HIV infection among males:		
ages 16-17	0.01%	0.13%
age 18	0.03%	0.29%
age 19	0.07%	0.55%
age 20	na	0.65%
Percent with HIV infection among females:		
ages 16-17	0.02%	0.22%
age 18	0.03%	0.35%
age 19	0.05%	0.23%
age 20	na	0.45%
HIV infection rates by Race and Ethnicity:		
White	0.02%	0.12%
African American	0.10%	0.53%
Hispanic	0.03%	0.26%

(k) Burke, D.S., et al. "Human Immunodeficiency Virus Infections in Teenagers: Seroprevalence Among Applicants for U.S. Military Service." Journal of the American Medical Association [JAMA]. Vol. 263. No. 15. 1990. p. 2074-2077.

St. Louis, M.E., et al. "Human Immunodeficiency Virus Infection in Disadvantaged Adolescents: Findings From the U.S. Job Corps." JAMA. Vol. 266. No. 17. November 1991. p. 2387-2391.

As indicated in Table 6, more than one in every 300 adolescents who entered the Job Corps during the study period was infected with HIV, compared with more than one in every 3,000 teenagers who applied for entry into military service. The tenfold difference in seroprevalence rates reflects differences in HIV prevalence in the populations sampled. The military sample was dominated by whites and high school graduates; the Job Corps sample consisted of predominantly disadvantaged minorities and high school dropouts. While drug addiction excludes applicants to both Job Corps and military service, the Job Corps does not exclude adolescents with a history of drug use, or who are homosexual and/or bisexual.[22]

Despite differences in populations, both studies found higher rates of HIV infection in African-American and Hispanic youth than in white youth. By age 21, nearly one in 80 minority entrants to the Job Corps was infected with HIV.[23]

The military and Job Corps studies also found that HIV infection rates were higher in females ages 16-18 than among males. In fact, the ratios of male-to-female infections were significantly lower than those found from AIDS case surveillance data, (1.1:1 and 1.2:1 in the military and the Job Corps studies respectively, compared with 2.7:1 in youth ages 13-19 diagnosed with AIDS).

C. DATA REGARDING SEXUAL BEHAVIORS AND DRUG USE AMONG ADOLESCENTS ALSO INDICATE THEY ARE AT RISK OF HIV INFECTION

Since the early 1970s, the incidence of sexually transmitted diseases (STDs), unintended pregnancy, and other problems associated with sexual activity have increased among adolescents in the United States.[24] For example, approximately one million adolescent females become pregnant each year. By 1989, birth rates for teenagers had increased to levels not observed for 15 years.[25] Additionally, 86% of all STDs occur among persons ages 15-29 years.[26] While not all teens are sexually active or drug users, available data indicate that many adolescents currently engage in sexual and drug use behaviors that put them at risk for HIV infection.

HIV infection.

For adolescents who have not had sexual intercourse and who have not shared needles or syringes, the risk of HIV infection is low. At higher risk are adolescents who:

- engage in sexual intercourse at early ages;
- have several sexual partners;
- have a sexually transmitted disease;
- practice intercourse without consistent and proper use of latex condoms with spermicide;
- engage in male-to-male sexual relations;
- engage in anal intercourse;
- inject drugs (including cocaine, amphetamines, steroids, and heroin);
- or who have sex with injecting drug users.[27]

As noted by the National Research Council in 1990, no single statistic captures the complex dimensions of risk or the considerable variation in the prevalence of sexual and drug use behaviors across all ages, genders, and racial subgroups.[28] However, research describing the prevalence of the above-mentioned behaviors among adolescents provides an alternative method of estimating their risk of HIV infection.

By age 20, 68% of adolescent females and 86% of adolescent males are sexually active. Two national surveys offer estimates of trends in adolescent sexual behavior: the 1988 National Survey of Family Growth (NSFG) and the 1988 National Survey of Adolescent Males (NSAM). During the past two decades, there has been a steady increase in both the proportion of young teens who are sexually active, and in the number of their premarital sexual partners.[29]

Greater Proportion of Adolescent Females Sexually Active, Age of First Intercourse Dropping

According to the NSFG study, the percent of females ages 15-19, who reported having engaged in sexual intercourse rose from 47% in 1982 to 53% in 1988.[30] As shown in Figure 2, much of the increase can be attributed to increases occurring among white and non-poor teens, thus narrowing racial and

Figure 2: Percent of Adolescent Females Ages 15-19 Who Ever Had Sexual Intercourse, By Race/Ethnicity and Poverty Level, 1982 and 1988[l]

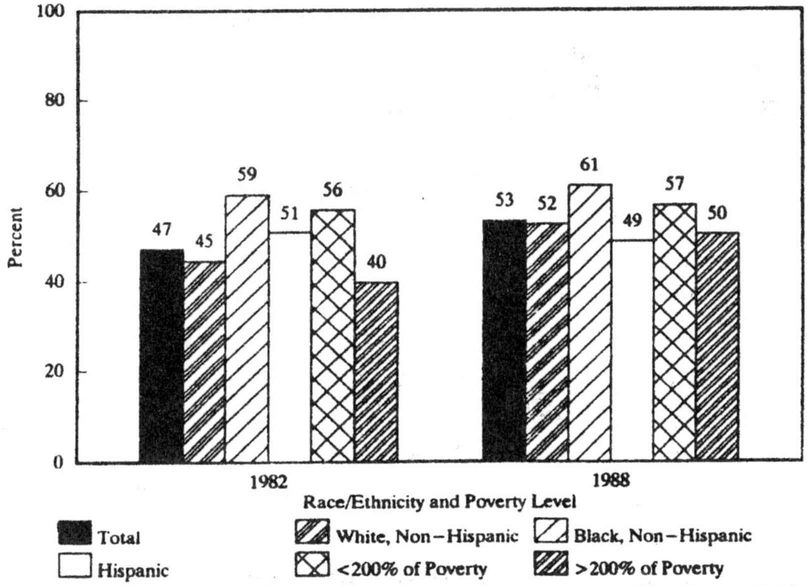

(l) Reprinted with the permission of The Alan Guttmacher Institute from Jacqueline Darroch Forrest and Susheela Singh, "The Sexual and Reproductive Behavior of American Women, 1982-1988." Family Planning Perspectives. Vol. 22. No. 5. September/October 1990.

Sexual activity increases dramatically with age among adolescent females. NSFG data tabulated by the National Research Council indicate that in 1988, 10% of females reported engaging in sexual intercourse before age 15; 35% reported intercourse before age 17; and nearly 70% of young women reported sexual intercourse before age 20.[32] (See Table 7)

Table 7: Percent of Never-Married Females Born Between 1964-1972 Who Report Engaging in Sexual Intercourse, By Age at First Intercourse and Race[(m)]

Age	All	African-American	White
Before 14	4.1%	8.0%	2.8%
Before 15	10.3%	17.4%	8.2%
Before 16	20.9%	31.2%	18.9%
Before 17	35.2%	50.4%	33.0%
Before 18	49.7%	65.8%	48.8%
Before 19	62.7%	80.7%	62.0%
Before 20	68.2%	87.7%	66.5%

Percent of Sexually Active Adolescent Males Also Rising

Rates of sexual activity are also increasing among adolescent males. NSAM data (of males living in metropolitan areas) indicate that the proportion of males who had intercourse by age 19 increased from 78% in 1979 to 86% in 1988.[33]

As shown in Figure 3, in 1988, 33% of males age 15 reported having engaged in premarital intercourse. Among 17-year-old men, the proportion who were sexually active doubled to 66%; for those age 19, 86% reported having engaged in premarital sexual intercourse.[34]

(m) Reprinted with permission from AIDS: The Second Decade, c.1990 by the National Academy of Sciences. Published by the National Academy Press, Washington, DC. Percentages not shown for Hispanic females because of small sample size.

Figure 3: Percent of Never-Married Males Ages 15-19 Who Have Had Sexual Intercourse, By Age, According to Race/Ethnicity, 1988[n]

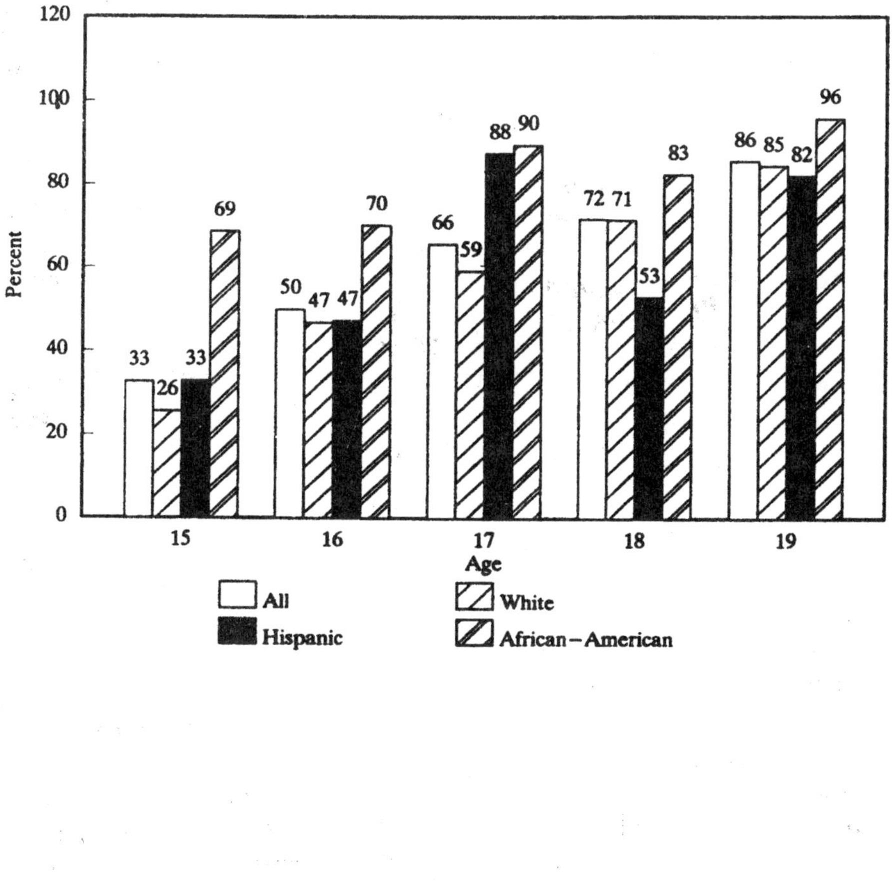

(n) Reprinted with the permission of The Alan Guttmacher Institute from Freya Sonenstein, Joseph Pleck, and Leighton C. Ku. "Sexual Activity, Condom Use and AIDS Awareness Among Adolescent Males." Family Planning Perspectives. Vol. 21. No. 4. July/August 1989.

Many Youth Report Multiple Sexual Partners

Once teens initiate sexual activity, many continue to engage in intercourse, often with multiple partners. Despite relatively short histories of sexual activity, 58% of sexually experienced females ages 15-19 reported having had sex with two or more partners. NSFG data also indicate that while nearly one-fourth of women ages 18-19 are not sexually active, almost the same proportion reported having had three to five partners and 11% reported having had six or more partners.[35]

Young men residing in metropolitan areas also reported numerous sexual partners. Nearly 20% of men ages 18-19 reported having had between three and five partners, and about the same proportion reported six to ten partners.[36]

One in Six Teens Affected by a Sexually Transmitted Disease Each Year, Prevalence of STDs Serves as Proxy for Sexual Risk Taking Among Youth

The aggregate annual costs of herpes, gonorrhea, chlamydia, and pelvic inflammatory disease are estimated to total $8.5 billion.[37] In 1980, a National Institute of Allergy and Infectious Diseases Study Group concluded that STDs were the most pervasive, destructive, and costly communicable diseases confronting adolescents.[38] Ten years later, the transmission of STDs in adolescents remains an urgent public health concern.

Adolescents are at higher risk for sexually transmitted infection than members of other age groups for a variety of behavioral, biological, and psychosocial reasons.[39] The CDC estimates that three million teens, or one in six, are affected by an STD annually and that nearly two-thirds of the more than 12 million STDs diagnosed in 1990 were among persons under age 25.[40] Left untreated, STDs may result in a number of serious health consequences including death, pelvic inflammatory disease, infertility, ectopic pregnancy, adverse pregnancy outcome, infant pneumonia, infant death, mental retardation, immune deficiencies, and neoplasia.[41] The prevalence of STDs in young adults is particularly troubling in light of recent studies showing that HIV transmission is enhanced when genital lesions from other STDs are present.[42]

No reliable sources of national data exist regarding STDs among adolescents.[43] Because states are not required to report various STDs, there is little uniformity in data collection about the prevalence and incidence of most sexually transmitted diseases.[44] Estimates of the prevalence of STDs are drawn from reportable disease registries, surveys of visits to office-based practices, data on patients attending specialized health facilities, and information gained from nationally representative samples of the population.[45]

STD rates among teens vary by sex and race, with more STDs reported among females than males, and among minority youth than whites. As noted by the Office of Technology Assessment (OTA) in its recent Adolescent Health report, differences between males and females may be explained in part because sexually active females are more likely than males to seek reproductive health care or family planning services where they may be screened for STDs. High STD rates among African-American and Hispanic youth may reflect the tendency of these adolescents, who are disproportionately from low-income families, to use public health clinics which report STDs more completely than private practitioners. Additionally, higher rates of sexual activity among African-American youth may account for higher rates of STDs in this population.[46]

As of March 1, 1989, only three states required reporting of chlamydia infections, the most common type of STD infection among adolescents.[47] Data from selected studies show that chlamydia infection rates vary from 3% to 37% depending on the surveyed population.[48] According to OTA, chlamydia infection has been found to be highly prevalent among certain subgroups of sexually active adolescents, particularly among African-American inner-city teenagers from low socioeconomic backgrounds. However, since the data are based on selected studies of teenagers attending various types of clinics, this finding may reflect the fact that many STD clinics are located in large metropolitan areas.[49]

All 50 states require reporting of gonorrhea and syphilis.[50] Because of the large number of cases reported every year, trends in gonorrhea provide the best estimates of STD patterns in teenagers.[51] During the 1980s, while gonorrhea rates declined in most age groups, they increased in males ages 15-19. Similarly, females ages 15-19 assumed the highest age-specific gonorrhea rate in 1984, and widened the gap over the next several years.[52] By 1989, more than one in four (29%) newly reported gonorrhea cases occurred among youth ages 10 to 19 years.[53]

Information about the prevalence of other STDs also indicate that significant numbers of adolescents may be at risk of HIV. In 1989, the most recent year for which data are available, the number of syphilis cases reported in the United States was at its highest level since World War II.[54] Between 1977 and 1987, the incidence rate of syphilis among females ages 10-14 and 15-19 increased approximately 120%. By 1989, nearly 10% of newly reported cases of syphilis were among persons ages 10-19.[55]

The most common consequence of STD infection for women is pelvic inflammatory disease (PID). Between 1975 and 1981, more than 260,000 women ages 15 to 44 experienced an episode of PID. Of these women, more than one in seven (16%) were teens ages 15 to 19 years. Nearly half (43%) of women hospitalized with PID are under age 25.[56]

Condom Use Increased During 1980s, Yet Many Adolescents Remain Unprotected From HIV and Other STDs

The most effective way to prevent infection from HIV and other STDs is to abstain from sexual intercourse. For those who are engaging in sexual intercourse, however, various studies among adults have found that correct and consistent use of latex condoms lubricated with the spermicide nonoxynol 9 provides an effective barrier to prevent transmission of STDs, including HIV.[57]

At hearings in June 1991 entitled: "The Risky Business of Adolescence: How to Help Teens Stay Safe," some Members of the Select Committee expressed concern that promoting condom use among sexually active adolescents could actually increase risk of HIV infection because condoms are not 100% effective.[58] Dr. Lloyd Kolbe, Director of the Division of Adolescent and School Health of the CDC, responded to these concerns. In collaboration with the Division of STD/HIV Prevention at CDC, Dr. Kolbe summarized the extensive body of research about condom effectiveness. His response included the following points:[59]

- When latex condoms are used consistently and correctly, they are extremely effective in preventing sexually transmitted diseases (STDs), including HIV.

- Although latex condoms have reduced the risk of contracting STDs in both laboratory and clinical studies, effectiveness has varied. Several studies show 100% effectiveness for latex condoms. The individual user, not the condom, is more likely to be responsible for any failure in protection from sexually transmitted infection or unwanted pregnancy.

- While the "typical" failure rate of condoms as contraceptives is approximately 10-20%, condom effectiveness as a contraceptive increases with experience, and failure rates as low as 0.6% have been documented.

- Manufacturing defects are quite uncommon. Each domestically manufactured condom is individually electronically tested for pinholes and areas of thinning, and imported batches are subject to testing by the Food and Drug Administration.

See Appendix C for materials submitted by Kolbe in response to concerns about condom effectiveness.

Between 1982 and 1988, the percent of teenage females practicing contraception rose significantly, from 24% to 32%, reflecting primarily an increase in condom use by this population.[60] In fact, the percent of females ages 15-19 who reported reliance on condoms for contraception increased from 21% in 1982 to 33% in 1988. During the same years, the percent of females relying on the pill for contraception decreased from 64% to 59%.[61]

The proportion of females ages 15-19 who reported *contraceptive use at first intercourse* also increased during the

1980s, from 48% in 1982 to 65% in 1988.[62] This increase was due principally to increased condom use reported by females of all races/ethnicities, and socioeconomic status.[63] (See Table 8)

Table 8: Percent of Sexually-Experienced Females Ages 15-19 Who Used Condoms and/or Any Method of Contraception at First Intercourse, By Race/Ethnicity, 1982 and 1988[(o)]

	1982		1988	
	Any Method	Condom Use	Any Method	Condom Use
Total	47.9%	22.6%	65.0%	47.4%
White, Non-Hispanic	54.6%	24.9%	69.0%	51.1%
Black, Non-Hispanic	35.8%	18.7%	54.1%	34.8%
Hispanic	22.5%	12.8%	53.9%	41.8%

Despite these improvements, it is important to note that more than one-third of females ages 15-19 do not use any method of contraception at first intercourse and that many young people, particularly females, delay contraceptive use for up to a year after first intercourse.[64]

Condom use among males has also increased significantly in the past decade. In 1979, 21% of sexually-active males ages 17-19 who were surveyed reported that they had used a condom *at last intercourse*. This figure rose to 58% in 1988.[65] As mentioned previously, condom use at *first intercourse* is especially important for HIV prevention, because younger teens tend to delay contraceptive use, including use of condoms, for many months or even years. Table 9 summarizes data reported by the 1988 National Survey of Adolescent Males.

(o) Reprinted with the permission of The Alan Guttmacher Institute from Jacqueline Darroch Forrest and Susheela Singh, "The Sexual and Reproductive Behavior of American Women, 1982-1988." Family Planning Perspectives. Vol. 22. No. 5. September/October 1990.

Table 9: Percent of Never-Married, Sexually-Active Males Ages 15-19, By Contraceptive Method Used At First Intercourse, According to Age at First Intercourse and Race/Ethnicity, 1988[(p)]

Method and Age at First Intercourse	All Races	White	African-American	Hispanic
Condoms Alone or With Other Methods				
all ages	55.0%	57.9%	43.5%	52.4%
<12	16.5%	2.2%	27.0%	11.8%
12-14	48.3%	52.3%	38.9%	41.9%
15-17	60.8%	61.5%	56.6%	59.5%
18-19	64.1%	63.7%	37.4%	66.1%
Ineffective or No Contraceptive Method				
all ages	37.8%	33.9%	50.6%	42.8%
<12	74.5%	70.8%	73.0%	88.2%
12-14	48.3%	44.6%	57.1%	53.0%
15-17	31.6%	30.6%	33.8%	36.0%
18-19	16.3%	15.1%	62.6%	11.4%

Homosexual Behavior May Be More Common in Teens than Previously Thought

As mentioned previously, although male homosexual behavior is implicated in a large number of AIDS cases among youth, a lack of reliable data has prevented accurate assessment of the prevalence of homosexual activity and risk-taking among adolescents who identify themselves as gay or lesbian.[66]

(p) Reprinted with the permission of The Alan Guttmacher Institute from Freya Sonenstein, Joseph Pleck, and Leighton C. Ku. "Sexual Activity, Condom Use and AIDS Awareness Among Adolescent Males." Family Planning Perspectives. Vol. 21. No. 4. July/August 1989.

In this table, effective methods of contraception include oral contraceptives, diaphragm, IUD, sponge, foam, jelly or suppository.

Since the Kinsey studies were conducted during the 1940s and 1950s, only one study using data from a national probability sample has estimated the prevalence of same-gender sex. This 1970 survey found that at least 20% of American men have had same-gender sexual contact to the point of orgasm, with the majority reporting that the first contact of this type occurred during their teenage years or earlier.[67]

Other smaller studies have confirmed that homosexual experimentation is more frequent among adolescents than commonly believed. One study of high school students in the Bronx found that 10% of female students and 9% of male students reported same-gender sex,[68] and four other surveys of young American men found that the incidence of homosexual activity resulting in orgasm on at least one occasion ranged from 17% to 37%.[69]

Homosexual activity during adolescence does not necessarily confirm a gay or lesbian sexual orientation, but it is important to note that many adolescents who may not consider themselves to be homosexual or bisexual, nevertheless participate in same-gender sexual behaviors that place them at risk of HIV infection.[70] (See Chapter III for further discussion of homosexual behavior among youth.)

Anal Intercourse Practiced by Heterosexual Adolescent Partners

Anal intercourse is particularly risky for HIV transmission because it may cause small tears in the rectal lining, which can allow infected semen to enter the bloodstream.[71] National estimates of the prevalence of this behavior are unavailable. However, one study found that more than one-fourth (25.2%) of teenage females attending an adolescent outpatient clinic in New York City reported having engaged in anal intercourse,[72] and another study found that of more than 100 females ages 15-21 interviewed at a family planning clinic, 12% reported that they had engaged in anal intercourse.[73]

Nearly One Million Teens Exchange Sex for Food, Shelter, Money, or Drugs

An estimated 150,000 adolescents become involved in prostitution each year,[74] and according to one study by the American Medical Association, an estimated 900,000 teens have exchanged sex for food, shelter, money, or drugs. Of these youth, two-thirds are female.[75]

Drug Use Prevalent Among Teens, Associated with Risky Sexual Behavior

Millions of young adults experiment with alcohol and other drug use each year. Although intravenous drug use is particularly risky in terms of HIV infection, other drugs can play a less direct role in HIV transmission because they can impair a user's judgment, leading the user to engage in higher risk sexual behaviors.[76]

Data from the 1991 National Household Survey and the 1990 National High School Senior Survey indicate that over four million young people ages 12-17 (20.1% of this population) have used an illicit drug at least one time during their lives; over 2.9 million (14.8%) have used an illicit drug within the past year, and nearly 1.4 million (6.8%) of young people ages 12-17 had used illicit drugs in the month prior to the interview. (See Table 10)

Table 10. Percent of Adolescents Ages 12 to 17 Reporting Drug Use, 1991[q]

	Ever Used	Used at Least Once In Previous Year
Any Illicit Drug	20.1%	14.8%
Marijuana	13.0%	10.1%
Inhalants	7.0%	4.1%
Hallucinogens	3.4%	2.1%
PCP	1.1%	0.6%
Cocaine	2.4%	1.5%
Crack	0.9%	0.4%
Heroin	0.3%	0.2%
Nonmedical Use of Psychotherapeutics	7.5%	5.4%
Stimulants	3.0%	1.9%
Sedatives	2.4%	1.3%
Tranquilizers	2.1%	1.3%
Alcohol	46.4%	40.3%
Steroids	0.6%	0.3%

Older teens are even more likely to report illicit drug use, as indicated by data from the National High School Senior Drug Survey in Table 11.

(q) U.S. Department of Health and Human Services, National Institute on Drug Abuse (NIDA). National Household Survey on Drug Abuse: Population Estimates 1991. 1991. Psychotherapeutics include use of prescription-type stimulant, sedative, tranquilizer, or analgesic, excluding over-the-counter drugs.

Table 11. Percent of High School Class of 1990 Reporting Drug Use[(r)]

	Ever Used	Used at Least Once In Previous Year
Marijuana	40.7%	27.0%
Inhalants	18.0%	6.9%
Hallucinogens	9.7%	5.9%
LSD	8.7%	5.4%
PCP	2.8%	1.2%
Cocaine	9.4%	5.3%
Crack	3.5%	1.9%
Heroin	1.3%	0.5%
Other Opiates	8.3%	4.5%
Stimulants	17.5%	9.1%
Sedatives	7.5%	3.6%
Tranquilizers	7.2%	3.5%
Alcohol	89.5%	80.6%
Steroids	2.9%	1.7%

In 1991, the Department of Health and Human Services reported that eight million junior and senior high school students (nearly 40% of this population) reported weekly consumption of alcohol, including 5.4 million students who had "binged" with five or more drinks in a row, and 454,000 who reported an average weekly consumption of 15 drinks.[77]

Adolescents who may be at highest risk of injecting drug use or risky sexual behavior related to alcohol or drug using behavior include youngsters who have engaged in prostitution, are runaways or are homeless, have been detained or incarcerated, or have been abused.[78]

It is important to note that the High School Senior Survey

(r) NIDA. Drug Use Among American High School Seniors, College Students and Young Adults, 1975-1990 - Vol. 1: High School Seniors. Rockville, MD. 1991. Percents for inhalants are not adjusted for known underreporting of amyl and butyl nitrates. Only drug use which was not under a doctor's orders is included for opiates, stimulants, sedatives, and tranquilizers.

included only adolescents who attended high school. However, drug use has been documented at significantly higher levels among certain segments of the teenage population, many of whom do not attend school.[79] Similarly, while the 1990 National Household Survey sample included adolescent school dropouts living at home and persons living in homeless shelters, it does not include runaways, transient populations (such as homeless youth not in shelters), or those who were detained or incarcerated.

Crack Use Linked To Spread of HIV

Crack (a smokable form of cocaine) is believed to play an important role in the HIV epidemic due to its highly addictive properties and its association with increases in an individual's sexual drive and subsequent increases in unprotected sexual activity.[80] According to the Chairman of the National Commission on AIDS, June Osborne, crack use is thought to have contributed to high levels of HIV and other STDs in a number of states including New York, New Jersey, and Georgia.[81]

A study of 222 African-American teenage crack users from San Francisco and Oakland found that 96% were sexually active, 62% had sold crack, 51% had combined crack use and sex, 41% reported a history of STDs, and 25% had exchanged sexual favors for drugs or money. While the average age of first intercourse was 12.8 years among the study population, the age at first condom use was 14.8 years.[82] (See Chapter III for further analysis of drug use among youth and its role in the HIV epidemic.)

Endnotes

1 Institute of Medicine. Report of a Study: The AIDS Research Program of the National Institutes of Health. Washington, D.C.: National Academy Press, 1991.

2 Conclusion by Select Committee based on the evidence presented in this chapter. Cites include the following: Miller, H.G., et al. (eds.) AIDS: The Second Decade. Washington, D.C.: National Academy Press. 1990; Novick, L.F., et al. "Newborn Seroprevalence Study: Methods and Results." American Journal of Public Health: New York State HIV Seroprevalence Project. Vol. 81. Supplement. May 1991; Burke, D.S., et al. "Human Immunodeficiency Virus Infections in Teenagers: Seroprevalence Among Applicants for U.S. Military Service." Journal of the American Medical Association. Vol. 263. No. 15. 1990; St.Louis, M.E., et al. "Human Immunodeficiency Virus Infection in Disadvantaged Adolescents: Findings From the U.S. Job Corps." Journal of the American Medical Association. Vol. 266. No. 17. 1991; U.S. Department of Health and Human Services, National Center for Health Statistics, (NCHS). "Advance Report of Final Natality Statistics, 1989." Monthly Vital Statistics Report: Final Data." Vol. 40. No. 8. Supplement. December 1991; U.S. Department of Health and Human Services, Public Health Service. Centers for Disease Control (CDC). "Sexual Behavior Among High School Students - United States, 1990." Morbidity and Mortality Weekly Report. Vol. 40. Nos. 51 and 52. January 1992; Forrest, J.D. and Singh, S. "The Sexual and Reproductive Behavior of American Women, 1982-1988." Family Planning Perspectives. Vol. 22. No. 5. September/October 1990; Sonenstein, F.L., et al. "Sexual Activity, Condom Use and AIDS Awareness Among Adolescent Males." Family Planning Perspectives. Vol. 21. No. 4. July/August 1989; CDC. Division of STD/HIV Prevention. Cates, W. [Former] Director. "The Epidemiology and Control of Sexually Transmitted Diseases in Adolescents." In Adolescent Medicine: State of the Art Reviews - Philadelphia, PA: Hanley and Belfus, Inc. Vol. 1. No. 3. October 1990; Mosher, W.D. "Contraceptive Practice in the United States, 1982-1988." Family Planning Perspectives. Vol. 22. No. 5. September/October 1990; Turner, C.F., et al. (eds.) AIDS, Sexual Behavior, and Intravenous Drug Use. Washington, D.C.: National Academy Press, 1989; Reuben, N., et al. "Relationships of High-risk Behaviors to AIDS Knowledge in Adolescent High School Students." Presented at the Annual

Research Meeting of the Society for Adolescent Medicine, New York City, March. (Cited by Miller, H.G., et al. (eds.) 1990. op cit.); Remafedi, G.J. "Preventing the Sexual Transmission of AIDS During Adolescence." Journal of Adolescent Health Care. Vol. 9. No. 2. March 1988; Jaffe, L.R., et al. "Anal Intercourse and Knowledge of Acquired Immunodeficiency Syndrome Among Minority-Group Female Adolescents." Journal of Pediatrics. Vol. 112. 1988. (Cited by Miller, H.G., et al. (eds.) 1990. op cit.); Kegeles, S., et al. "AIDS Risk Behavior Among Sexually Active Hispanic and Caucasian Adolescent Females." Presented at the Fifth International Conference on AIDS, Montreal, June 4-9, 1989. (As Reported in Miller, H.G., et al. (eds.) 1990. op cit.); U.S. Department of Health and Human Services, National Institute on Drug Abuse [NIDA]. National Household Survey on Drug Abuse: Population Estimates 1991. 1991; NIDA. Drug Use Among American High School Seniors, College Students and Young Adults, 1975-1990 - Vol. 1: High School Seniors. Rockville, MD. 1991; Fullilove, R.E., et al. "Crack Users: The New AIDS Risk Group?" Cancer Detection and Prevention. Vol. 14. Issue 3. 1990.

3 Peterman, T.A. and Petersen, L.R. "Stalking the Epidemic: Which Tracks to Follow and How Far?" American Journal of Public Health. Vol. 80. No. 4. April 1990.

4 Miller, H.G., et al. (eds.) 1990. op cit.

5 Peterman and Petersen. 1990. op cit.

6 Peterman and Petersen. 1990. op cit.

7 Miller, H.G., et al. (eds.) 1990. op cit.

8 Conway, G.A., et al. "Under-reporting of AIDS Cases in South Carolina, 1986 and 1987." Journal of the American Medical Association. Vol. 262. No. 20. 1989; CDC. "Understanding AIDS: An Information Brochure Being Mailed to All U.S. Households." Morbidity and Mortality Weekly. Vol. 38. No. 17. 1989. (Cited by U.S. Congress. Office of Technology Assessment [OTA]. Adolescent Health - Volume II: Background and The Effectiveness of Selected Prevention and Treatment Services. Washington, D.C.: Government Printing Office. November 1991.)

9 Miller, H.G., et al. (eds.) 1990. op cit.; Hein, K. Personal Communication. March 10, 1992.

10 CDC. "1992 Revised Classification System for HIV Infection and Expanded AIDS Surveillance Case Definition for Adolescents and Adults." November 15, 1991; CDC. "Review of Draft for Revision of HIV Infection Classification System and Expansion of AIDS Case Surveillance Definition." Morbidity and Mortality Weekly Report. Vol. 40. No. 45. 1991; "Redefining AIDS Would Add 160,000 Cases." The Washington Post. Washington, D.C. November 15, 1991.)

11 Hein, K. Montefiore Medical Center, Department of Pediatrics. New York, NY. Personal Communication. March 10, 1992.

12 CDC. "HIV/AIDS Surveillance, Year End Edition, U.S. Cases Reported through December 1991." January 1992; CDC. "HIV/AIDS Surveillance, Year-End Edition, U.S. Cases Reported Through December 1990." January 1991.

13 OTA. November 1991. op cit.

14 CDC. "HIV/AIDS Surveillance, Year End Edition, U.S. Cases Reported through December 1991." January 1992. op cit.

15 CDC. "HIV Prevalence Estimates and AIDS Case Projections for the United States: Report Based Upon a Workshop." Morbidity and Mortality Weekly Report. Vol. 39. No. RR-16. November 1990.

16 Miller, H.G., et al. (eds.) 1990. op cit.

17 Miller, H.G., et al. (eds.) 1990. op cit.; OTA. November 1991. op cit.

18 Miller, H.G., et al. (eds.) 1990. op cit.

19 Novick, L.F., et al. 1991. op cit.

20 Miller, H.G., et al. (eds.) 1990. op cit.

21 Burke, D.S., et al. 1990. op cit.; St.Louis, M.E., et al. 1991. op cit.

22 DiClemente, R.J. "Epidemiology of AIDS, HIV Prevalence and HIV Incidence Among Adolescents." (in press.) Used with Permission.

23 St. Louis, M.E., et al. 1991. op cit.

24 CDC. Morbidity and Mortality Weekly Report. January 1992. op cit.

25 NCHS. 1991. op cit.

26 CDC. Morbidity and Mortality Weekly Report. November 1992. op cit.

27 OTA. 1991. op cit.

28 Miller, H.G., et al. (eds.) 1990. op cit.

29 Miller, H.G., et al. (eds.) 1990. op cit.; Turner, C.F., et al. (eds.) 1989. op cit.

30 Forrest, J.D. and Singh, S. 1990. op cit.

31 Forrest, J.D. and Singh, S. 1990. op cit.

32 Miller, H.G., et al. (eds.) 1990. op cit.

33 Sonenstein, F.L., et al. 1989. op cit.

34 Sonenstein, F.L., et al. 1989. op cit.

35 Forrest, J.D. and Singh, S. 1990. op cit.

36 Miller, H.G., et al. (eds.) 1990. op cit.

37 CDC. Division of STD/HIV Prevention. Annual Report. 1990.

38 DiClemente, R.J. "Commentary - Prevention of HIV Among Adolescents: The Interplay of Health Education and Public Policy in the Development and Implementation of School-Based AIDS Education Programs." AIDS Education and Prevention. Vol. 1. No. 1. 1989.

39 CDC. October 1990. op cit.

40 CDC. Division of STD/HIV Prevention. Annual Report. 1990. op cit.

41 CDC. Division of STD/HIV Prevention. Annual Report. 1990. op cit.

42 Miller, H.G., et al. (eds.) 1990. op cit.; CDC. October 1990. op cit.

43 OTA. Adolescent Health - Volume I: Summary and Policy Options. Washington, D.C.: Government Printing Office. April 1991.

44 OTA. November 1991. op cit.

45 CDC. October 1990. op cit.

46 OTA. November 1991. op cit.

47 OTA. November 1991. op cit.

48 OTA. November 1991. op cit.

49 OTA. November 1991. op cit.

50 OTA. November 1991. op cit.

51 CDC. October 1990. op cit.

52 CDC. October 1990. op cit.

53 OTA. April 1991. op cit.

54 CDC. October 1990. op cit.

55 OTA. April 1991. op cit.

56 OTA. November 1991. op cit.

57 Kolbe, L.J. CDC. Written testimony submitted for hearing, The Risky Business of Adolescence: How To Help Teens Stay Safe. Select Committee on Children, Youth, and Families, U.S. House of Representatives. Washington, D.C. June 17, 1991; OTA. November 1991. op cit.

58 Jones, E.F. and Forrest, J.D. "Contraceptive Failure Rates Based on the 1988 NSFG." Family Planning Perspectives. Vol. 24. No. 1. January/February 1992; Trussell, J., et al. "Condom Slippage

and Breakage Rates." Family Planning Perspectives. Vol. 24. No. 1. January/February 1992.

59 Kolbe, L.J. June 1991. op cit.

60 Mosher, W.D. 1990. op cit.

61 Mosher, W.D. 1990. op cit.

62 Forrest, J.D. and Singh, S. 1990. op cit.

63 Forrest, J.D. and Singh, S. 1990. op cit.

64 OTA. November 1991. op cit.

65 Sonenstein, F.L., et al. 1989. op cit.

66 Turner, C.F., et al. (eds.) 1989. op cit.

67 Miller, H.G., et al. (eds.) 1990. op cit.

68 Reuben, N., et al. 1990. op cit.

69 Remafedi, G.J. 1988. op cit.

70 Miller, H.G., et al. (eds.) 1990. op cit.; American Academy of Pediatrics, Committee on Adolescence. "Homosexuality and Adolescence." Pediatrics. 1983.

71 Remafedi, G.J. "Fundamental Issues in the Care of Homosexual Youth." Medical Clinics of North America. Vol. 74. No. 5. September 1990.

72 Jaffe, L.R., et al. 1988. op cit.

73 Kegeles, S., et al. 1989. op cit.

74 Millstein, S. "AIDS in the Adolescent Population: A High Risk Group in Urgent Need of Preventive Education." Carnegie Council on Adolescent Development. March 1988. (Cited by AIDS Action Foundation. "HIV and Adolescents -- Final, Final Draft." January 20, 1990.)

75 American Medical Association (AMA). White Paper on Adolescent Health. Chicago, IL: AMA. 1986. (Cited by Center

for Population Options. "Out of the Shadows: Building an Agenda and Strategies for Preventing HIV/AIDS in Street and Homeless Youth." Washington, D.C. 1990.)

76 Flavin, D.K. and Frances, R.J. "Risk Taking Behavior, Substance Abuse Disorders, and the Acquired Immunodeficiency Syndrome." Advances in Alcohol and Substance Abuse. Vol. 6. 1987; Miller, H.G., et al. (eds.) 1990. op cit.

77 U.S. Department of Health and Human Services, Office of the Inspector General. Youth and Alcohol: A National Survey. June 1991.

78 OTA. November 1991. op cit.

79 OTA. November 1991. op cit.

80 Fullilove, R.E., et al. 1990. op cit.; CDC. October 1990. op cit.; Miller, H.G., et al. (eds.) 1990. op cit.

81 Osborne, J.E., Dean, School of Public Health, University of Michigan, Ann Arbor, MI. Personal Communication with OTA, as reported in OTA. November 1991. op cit.

82 Fullilove, R.E., et al. "Risk of Sexually Transmitted Diseases Among Black Adolescent Crack Users in Oakland and San Francisco California." Journal of the American Medical Association. Vol. 263. 1990.

CHAPTER II

PREVENTING RISKY BEHAVIOR IN ADOLESCENTS†

There is no preventive vaccine or cure for AIDS, so eliminating risky behavior that might lead to HIV infection is the only way to stop the spread of the virus.[1] Effective HIV prevention programs for adolescents must dispel myths, impart knowledge about HIV transmission and self-protection, reinforce or instill health promoting attitudes and behaviors, and, ultimately lead to sustained avoidance of high-risk behavior.[2]

Few HIV prevention programs for adolescents have been rigorously evaluated. Some interventions have increased knowledge about AIDS or even induced reported changes in relevant attitudes. Unfortunately, responses on paper in a classroom do not guarantee reductions in high-risk behavior or increases in health-promoting behavior.[3]

HIV prevention programs have adopted promising strategies from efforts to reduce smoking and other risky behaviors common among teenagers. Additional HIV prevention program guidance has emerged from the front-line experience of educators, public health officials and youth service providers.[4]

Even if a cure for HIV infection is found, prevention will continue to be necessary. New treatments will bring with them complex issues of experimentation with human subjects and problems with resource allocation. As the rise in the rate of syphilis infection has shown, no single intervention, even effective treatment, is likely to totally eradicate this major public health problem.[5]

A. COMPREHENSIVE HIV PREVENTION PROGRAMS MOST PROMISING

During the past several years, many efforts to reduce or eliminate the risk of HIV infection have been undertaken. Prevention campaigns targeting teenagers are underway in classrooms, school-based and community-based health clinics, other community settings, and the media.[6]

† Excerpted from CRS Report 102-1074

Program elements range from individualized counseling to comic books. Some programs employ a single type of intervention, while others utilize various combinations of strategies.[7]

The Select Committee on Children, Youth, and Families held hearings in June 1991, The Risky Business of Adolescence: How to Help Teens Stay Safe, to identify effective strategies for preventing risky behavior in adolescents. Several witnesses at the hearings pointed out that "AIDS 101" is insufficient to elicit behavior change in teenagers.

William Gardner of the University of Pittsburgh School of Medicine listed some of the necessary components of effective programs in his testimony to the Committee:

- Preventive education should begin early, before risk-taking behaviors begin;
- The intervention must be persistent, with messages delivered through many channels;
- The intervention should be comprehensive, addressing all adolescent risk-taking behaviors;
- The intervention should include social skills training to help the adolescent cope with peer cultural support for risk-taking; and,
- When adolescents are already participating in high-risk behavior, they need access to health services and intensive, individualized attention.[8] (See Chapter III)

Further direction for prevention programs comes from a report issued by the Committee on AIDS Research and the Behavioral, Social, and Statistical Sciences of the Institute of Medicine (IOM). The Committee found that HIV prevention programs should disseminate clear, specific information to all adolescents about the dangers of drug use and unprotected sex, and about the protective value of abstinence, condoms and spermicides. Adolescents at highest risk should be (1) provided special outreach and information, (2) aided in altering the behaviors that put them at risk, and (3) offered assistance in escaping the social or economic conditions that foster risk-taking.[9] This guidance was recently reiterated by the Office of Technology Assessment (OTA).[10]

Several sets of guidelines for HIV prevention programs for adolescents are available. References for guidelines are listed in Appendix C of this report, and include those developed by the Centers for Disease Control (CDC) and others tailored to address special needs such as those of young people in rural schools. Chapter III provides descriptions of model programs targeting specific populations.

B. LESSONS FROM TEEN PREGNANCY PREVENTION APPLY

Because few evaluations of HIV prevention programs for teens have been conducted to date,[11] existing information about preventing other problems associated with high-risk behaviors must guide HIV prevention programmers.[12] Certain program components have been shown to be necessary to prevent any type of undesirable outcome of high-risk sexual behavior in this age group, and program design must take into account the psychological realities of adolescence.[13]

No Single Solution: Education, Communication With Adults, Skills Training and Health Care Access All Needed to Reduce Pregnancy

The Office of Adolescent Pregnancy (OAP) has funded abstinence promotion over the last ten years.[14] Studies of the impact of a single "Just Say No" approach to teen pregnancy prevention show that it does not actually change behavior, and may ignore important adolescent characteristics.[15]

Kathleen Sullivan, Director of Project Respect in Illinois, reported statistically significant differences in teens' reported beliefs and attitudes about sex after participation in her abstinence promotion program. For example, "When asked, 'Are sexual urges controllable?' 28% said 'Always' on the pre-test in this past year and that went up to 48% on the post test."[16]

However, formal evaluations of the program show no evidence of behavior change in Project Respect participants.[17]

By contrast, abstinence programs that add social skills training (including topics such as assertiveness, refusal skills, interpersonal problem solving, and decision making) which are taught by high status individuals (e.g., respected peers) have resulted in as much as one year's postponement of sexual initiation in young teens (8th and 9th graders).[18] However, even the most successful abstinence programs have had little effect on the behavior of older teens who were already sexually active and therefore at higher risk of both pregnancy and HIV.[19]

Similarly, traditional school-based sex education alone, while necessary, appears insufficient to reduce the prevalence of unprotected sex. At the "Risky Business" hearing, Bradley P. Hayton cited evidence in his written testimony that sex education (in the absence of skills training, mentoring and health care access) has not been shown to delay sexual activity or to increase use of contraception.[20]

However, broader approaches that supplement education with certain additional services have proved effective with many older teenagers. A level of funding characteristic of multi-mode programs is required to "...provide ample dosage to offset this major socio-cultural problem."[21]

Demonstration programs such as <u>The School/Community Program for Sexual Risk Reduction Among Teens</u>, designed by Professor Murray Vincent of the School of Public Health of the University of South Carolina,[22] and <u>Preventing Adolescent Pregnancy</u>, by Girls' Inc.[23] have shown that teen pregnancy rates can be cut by more than one-third when several key program elements are combined. Effective demonstration programs comprised health care services (including contraceptive access or distribution), individual counseling, career planning, social skills training, parent/child communication workshops, and sexuality or family life education.[24]

It should be noted that, even when comprehensive programs have demonstrated effectiveness at one point in time, continual monitoring and constant readjustments of program quality are necessary to maintain momentum. A case in point is the South Carolina example mentioned above -- pregnancy rates climbed back to original levels three years after the intervention when access to contraceptive services was reduced and trained teachers left the school system.[25]

Program planners in Maryland, recently named the model state in adolescent pregnancy prevention by the Southern Governors' Association, have deemed comprehensive services the most promising approach. At the June hearings, Bronwyn Mayden, Executive Director of Maryland's Governor's Council on Adolescent Pregnancy, offered a partial explanation for the need for comprehensive services:

> Different strategies are needed [because] adolescents are not a monolith....Teen pregnancy is a complex phenomenon involving concepts of personal worth and identity, social norms and pressures, the allure of taking pleasure while avoiding responsibility, and economic deprivation. This complexity demands a comprehensive response.[26]

Gardner also emphasized this point in the context of HIV prevention:

> At present, efforts to reduce risky behaviors among adolescents are failing....The primary cause of this failure is the use of one-shot, educational efforts, where intensive, long-term programs are required.[27]

In summary, it is not unusual for adolescents to exhibit an increase in knowledge, or to report changes in their attitudes about sex as a result of participation in a single-mode intervention. However, teens appear to alter behavior patterns only if they receive a repeated, consistent message, develop the skills to make use of it, and have support for change from groups with whom they identify.[28] Generally, in order to display marked effects of training, youth must participate in the majority of the sessions in a prevention curriculum,[29] and have access to necessary health services. Individual attention from adults appears to be particularly important for youth at high risk.[30]

C. AIDS RISKS AND OTHER RISKS ARE RELATED

Adolescents who are prone to take risks often exhibit more than one kind of risky behavior.[31] Thus, strategies shown to be successful in preventing smoking, drug abuse and other sexually transmitted diseases in adolescents may well apply to HIV prevention.[32]

For example, studies of smoking cessation programs have shown that attempts to frighten teenagers are not particularly effective, and can sometimes backfire.[33] Interventions designed to prevent HIV infection should convince young people that they can become infected, while not raising anxiety levels to the point of creating denial, hopelessness, or negative effects on sexual development.[34]

In turn, effective HIV prevention programs should lower the prevalence of other problems caused by the same high-risk sexual and drug use behaviors that transmit HIV infection.[35] Several witnesses at the June hearings told the Committee that narrowly targeted preventive efforts (such as the Drug Free School Program of the Department of Education) should be broadened to address other HIV-related risks.[36]

Lloyd Kolbe, Director of the Division of Adolescent and School Health (DASH) of the CDC, advised the Committee that it would not be difficult to develop prevention techniques that address interrelated risks, noting that "CDC has designed its current program principally to prevent behaviors that result in HIV among youth...[but] it can be adapted to address other priority risk behaviors."[37]

Experience in school settings suggests an expansion of the focus of HIV prevention programs to other health-related behaviors wherever possible. Testimony submitted by the Human Rights Campaign Fund tracked the evolution of a model preventive program targeting gay and lesbian youth in the Los Angeles schools:

> ...into a general counseling and educational vehicle for both the gay and non-gay school population. The Project 10

> model provides for education, school safety, drop-out prevention strategies, and support services.[38]

Research in a variety of settings has documented the success of a comprehensive approach to prevention of high-risk behavior. Joy Dryfoos, author of a recent book reviewing the adolescent risk prevention literature, has pointed out that:

> The most successful programs [appear] to be focused on the underlying problems of youth, rather than simply the categorical behaviors such as using substances, being involved in precocious sexual behavior or being truant.[39]

Underlying problems that Dryfoos found predictive of high-risk behavior include: a lack of basic skills or of parental support; little ability to resist peer pressure; living in a disadvantaged community; and, feelings of depression and stress.

D. KNOWLEDGE OF ADOLESCENT PSYCHOLOGICAL DEVELOPMENT CRITICAL TO PROGRAM DESIGN

Taking the psychological development of teens into account when designing HIV prevention programs for this population presents considerable challenges, but it is essential that they be addressed. Adolescent psychology has been characterized by its strong orientation to peer culture, illusions of personal invulnerability, and natural tendency towards risk-taking.[40]

Dorothy Wodraska, a witness at the Select Committee's June prevention hearings from Project I-STAR (Indiana Students Taught Awareness and Resistance), a drug prevention program with demonstrated effectiveness in changing adolescent behavior, explained that middle school is a prime point for intervention because:

> ...young people are more susceptible to peer influence at this time compared to other stages in their development and are at greatest risk for beginning experimentation. Early adolescence is a high-risk period for young people, also the one most amenable to change and the one most associated with prevention of onset [of risky behavior].[41]

Furthermore, young adolescents' thinking tends to be concrete and egocentric, and not to be future-oriented. Two important skills increase during adolescence: The ability to anticipate the consequences of one's actions, and the ability to integrate specific facts into a general, coherent framework.[42] Future consequences and implications of specific behaviors should be clearly articulated in teen-oriented prevention programs.[43]

There is also evidence that children and adolescents use decision rules different from those of adults in making moral judgments.[44] Thus, forcing one limited version of morality on teenagers not only ignores the diversity in moral positions adults hold (a misrepresentation teens are likely to discern),[45] but may also prove futile because of the way teenagers think.[46]

Optimally, all adolescents should be developing self-control and the ability to form mature intimate relationships.[47] From one point of view, then, making decisions about substance use and sexual experimentation can serve to fulfill basic developmental needs.[48] Ironically, this "normal" behavior can have life threatening consequences. An HIV prevention instructor's credibility can hinge on acknowledging the contradictions in society's messages to adolescents.[49]

E. HOW TO DELIVER CRITICAL AIDS MESSAGES

Experts recommend that certain specific facts should be imparted in HIV prevention classes, such as the relative superiority of latex over lambskin condoms in blocking transmission of the virus.[50] However, the most important single message for adolescents may be: "It is not who you are, but what you do that places you at risk of AIDS." Emphasizing risk groups to teens can lead to self-labeling as immune. When the HIV virus is present, needle sharing among athletes using steroids can be just as deadly as unprotected sex with an IV drug user.[51]

Different aspects of a prevention message will be salient to teens at different ages. If information from smoking prevention program evaluations can be generalized, it is likely that physical aspects of the disease will be more meaningful to 12-year-olds, and that the social and psychological aspects will increase in importance with age.[52] Descriptions of immediate effects of high-risk behavior should be more compelling to adolescents than long-range impact.[53]

The OTA Adolescent Health report advised that the way information is transmitted may be important in students' ability to retain new knowledge. The OTA review provided support for multi-media presentations, active participation, and the use of role models to alter misconceptions and inoculate against media influences.[54]

Even when programmers take care to present essential information in the best possible form for a specific age group, information alone may not be sufficient to prevent high-risk behavior. Knowledge gains do not guarantee change in general attitudes, intentions to change specific behaviors, or change in high-risk behavior itself.[55]

OTA illustrated the limited value of information alone with the finding that, although most students know that condoms will help protect them, less than half of all adolescents who are sexually active use condoms, and only half of those who use them do so all the time. Moreover, perceived risk of AIDS did not predict condom use in a sample of adolescents at a family planning clinic in Baltimore,[56] or in runaways in New York City.[57] A dramatic increase in condom use was noted, however, when the full range of needs of a group of runaways was addressed by a comprehensive demonstration program.[58]

While research supports the recommendations made above, an important caution emerges from the same scientific literature. Well designed prevention programs (such as smoking cessation efforts) targeting adolescents have been somewhat successful with white, middle-class youth. However, with rare exceptions such as a recent project sponsored by the Rand Corporation,[59] most evaluations have failed to demonstrate behavior change in minority youth. It may be possible to strengthen prevention programs for minority youth by finding out more about perceived meanings of high-risk behavior as they vary by gender, ethnicity, and social demographics. Involving parents and peers in the design of prevention programs should be useful in this respect, as in other design considerations.[60] (See Chapter III "HIV-Related Needs of Racial and Ethnic Minority Adolescents.")

F. SCHOOLS AND COMMUNITIES PLAY KEY ROLES

K-12 "Healthy School" Programs Offer a Prime Context For HIV Prevention Efforts

The majority of young adolescents (more than 45 million) are in school, so schools are logical settings for prevention programming.[61] Only 31 states and the District of Columbia had mandated HIV education programming in the schools as of June 1991.[62] However, states such as Wisconsin have been very active in HIV education without a direct mandate. Conversely, mandates that were inadequately funded and lacking in political support have not resulted in strong local programming.[63] A large-scale response from every state is needed because cases of AIDS in adolescents or young adults have been reported in every state except North Dakota.[64]

The U.S. Department of Health and Human Services (DHHS) has taken the position that preventive HIV education would prove most effective if it were launched within the context of broader efforts to motivate health promotion and disease prevention.[65] Especially promising are the "healthy school" K-12 programs,[66] in which health-promoting behaviors are taught, health services are accessible, health-promoting environments are maintained, and attitudes that support healthy behavior are inculcated from an early age.[67]

One curriculum, Growing Healthy, has produced significant reductions in self-reported risk behaviors in high school students.[68] The Administration's national health objectives include establishing such sequential, K-12 health curricula in 75% of the nation's schools by the year 2000.[69]

A distinction should be drawn between comprehensive healthy school programs and school-based or school-linked health clinic services. The comprehensive healthy school model includes: (1) planned, sequential K-12 school health education; (2) health services; (3) a healthy and safe school environment; (4) physical education; (5) healthy school food service selections; (6) psychological assessment and counseling; (7) school site health promotion for faculty and staff; and, (8) integrated school and community health promotion efforts.[70] School-linked clinics are designed to provide access to the health services and counseling that are necessary within the larger healthy school model.[71]

Some states are attempting to initiate these comprehensive programs while simultaneously addressing the problem of teen access to health care. Testimony to the Committee provided by Lenore Zedosky, Assistant Director for the Office of Educational Support Services, West Virginia Department of Education, revealed that:

> Forty-seven of the 55 counties in West Virginia are designated as medically underserved areas....as students become more responsible for their own health and well-being, they must have access to health services that complement the health education program. Health centers will be located in schools to provide cost-effective, comprehensive services for students of all ages.[72]

According to a task force report submitted for the record of the June hearing by Governor Gaston Caperton of West Virginia:

> West Virginia can show significant improvement in the health status of its citizens by establishing progressive comprehensive school health programs. Communities, businesses and individuals will all benefit from these collaborative efforts. Healthy young people will become better educated, more productive and be far less likely to need premature, costly social and health services.[73]

Testimony submitted to the Committee by the American Academy of Pediatrics sounded an alarm regarding the extent of health and health care access problems experienced by teenagers throughout the United States:

> Teenagers and young adults represent the only segment of the United States population for whom mortality has risen over the past quarter century....The rate of adolescent mortality is the highest in the industrialized world...obstacles to health services...are both financial and geographic...adolescents are

> likelier than is any other age group to be uninsured or under-insured for health care services.[74]

A witness at the June hearings, Linda Dianne Meloy, noted that:

> In the face of all these risks, each adolescent needs a medical home to teach prevention, provide medical care, and to support appropriate development. A medical home must supply health instruction to the adolescent and their parents, medical care for the acute illnesses and chronic problems, counseling, phone service, and <u>easy access</u> twenty-four hours a day. I believe this expertise is found not in a clinic, but in the pediatrician's office and feel that every adolescent requires this care.[75]

The Academy of Pediatrics statement agreed that, ideally, every adolescent should have such a "medical home," but went on to explain that:

> Unfortunately, in many areas of our country, both urban and rural, this model of care is still unavailable. It is beyond debate that (in these special circumstances of physician scarcity) alternatives should be developed to fill the vacuum. Among such alternatives would certainly be school-based health care, which seeks to provide an impressive complement of services (logically) within the environment in which the adolescent is to be found.[76]

School-linked clinics increase teenagers' access to HIV-relevant health services (such as STD diagnosis and treatment), and offer counseling that may be prerequisite to heeding HIV prevention messages for young people at high risk. (See Chapter IV.) As a central component of comprehensive school health programs, health services have the potential to elicit behavior change in many students. Witnesses urged Congress to consider supporting comprehensive school health programs despite their initial cost because, over time, an investment in healthy schools should prove to be extremely sound in both human and financial terms.[77]

The imminent threat of HIV infection in adolescents has spurred a few communities to initiate school-based condom distribution programs. While some of these programs were added to ongoing health services and/or education, a handful were implemented in the absence of more comprehensive programs and are too new to assess for effectiveness.[78]

Parent/Community/School Partnerships Are Needed

Too often, AIDS educators try only to reach adolescents themselves in order to create and maintain incentives for individual behavior change in teenagers. According to a noted expert on adolescent risk-taking, Lewis P. Lipsitt, Executive Director for Science of the American Psychological Association, others must reinforce what the adolescents learn in school.[79]

Parents, teachers, peers, and the wider community play key roles in influencing the behavior of teenagers. All of these individuals and groups must learn more about the problem and participate actively in its solution to make preventive education fully effective.[80]

Parents have a special role to play in educating their children about HIV and AIDS. Involving parents reinforces information about HIV, its transmission and its prevention.[81] Successful involvement does not just happen: For example, workshops for parents may be needed to help them overcome widespread hesitancy to talk to teens about matters related to sex. In testimony before the Select Committee on Children, Youth, and Families, Robert Selverstone, President of the Sex Information and Education Council of the U.S. (SIECUS), explained that parents often feel they lack an appropriate vocabulary for talking about sex, doubt that their relevant knowledge is adequate, are habitually private about sexual matters, and fear value conflicts and confrontations with their children.[82]

In submitted testimony describing a multi-site, abstinence-oriented intervention attended by more than 3,000 participants, Mercedes Arzu Wilson offered support for the value of communication skills workshops for parents and youth:

> ...an evaluation and summary of the project was drawn up by two professors at the University of New Orleans. At the end

of the study, the evaluators concluded that the majority of parents responding to the Communication Skills questionnaire agreed that they had become more confident in their ability to discuss sexual concerns with their children following the workshops, and that they would likely engage in such discussions more frequently than prior to the workshops. Adolescents tended to perceive their parents as better sources of information regarding sexual matters than they were prior to program participation. Furthermore, responses of both parents and adolescents to pre- and post-project discussion forms indicated that the frequency of parent/adolescent conversations concerning human sexuality had increased subsequent to training.[83]

Communities in which parents have been involved from the outset in developing curricula are generally supportive of HIV prevention programming.[84] Testimony from the Human Rights Campaign Fund included survey results showing that the majority of parents support comprehensive HIV education:

> A recent survey by the Roper Organization found that an overwhelming majority of Americans believe that children as young as 12 should receive information about AIDS from their schools....While the majority of Americans understand that sexual abstinence is an effective way for a youth to remain HIV-negative, only one in seven believes that abstinence is a realistic solution to HIV transmission.[85]

Zedosky also emphasized the importance of involving other segments of the community:

> To be effective, wellness and disease prevention programs must be conducted in partnership with parents and the community....[In this way] School programs will be closely integrated with the existing service structure and social organization of the community.[86]

Zedosky listed several advantages of community participation in prevention programming, including opportunities for information exchange, social support, community "ownership" of the program, addressing health problems in context, and institutionalization of disease prevention and health promotion.

Community participation also expands prevention programming resources.[87] This expansion can occur through in-kind contributions, volunteer staff, resource sharing, technical assistance and financial investment. An illustration of what private sector organizations can add is the contribution to HIV education made by the Kaiser Permanente Health Maintenance Organization. This HMO has commissioned a health educational theater presentation for teens in six of its 12 regions, and produces the play in schools throughout the school year.

Joe Glosson, Director of Kaiser's Mid-Atlantic States Educational Theater Program, described the production to the Committee as follows:

> The SECRETS program is intended to increase student awareness of HIV and its transmission; reduce apprehension and prejudice arising from misinformation; and dispel myths and fears surrounding AIDS....SECRETS follows the story of Eddie and Monica, teenagers who must deal with their sexuality. Eddie has recently been involved in "risky behavior." Monica and a chain of other people figure in his journey from infection with HIV to living with the knowledge of a positive result. The play shows teenagers developing decision-making skills for resisting peer pressure, discussing choices with friends, and communicating with parents.
>
> Each 45 minute performance is followed by a question-and-answer session which is led by the actors, who receive extensive HIV/AIDS information training prior to the tour....Since February 1989 SECRETS has been performed 1,119 times to 614,000 students in 737 locations.[88]

Nonprofit community-based organizations have also played key roles in adolescent HIV prevention. A 15-year-old representative from the "Terrific Peers" program, Kianga Stroud, spoke to the Committee about the program's peer education efforts:

> Our program, Terrific Peers, believes that teens educating teens about AIDS is effective, and we strongly recommend it as one method....We communicate our message through role plays, raps and straight talk. I believe the message is better received by the teens we are trying to educate because

> we are teens also, not adults. We are on the same level. Also, our peers are impressed that we have so much information to share and are able to articulate it....I never participated in sex, drugs or any other risky behaviors but "Peers" has helped me to make the decision to continue to abstain from risky behavior.[89]

Another member of "Terrific Peers" described her preparation for educating peers to the Committee:

> My name is Eleshia Ray, I am 15 years old....I know what you are thinking, "What qualifies her to be an AIDS educator?" Well, we all received between 40-45 hours of training which we took over a period of five Saturdays. I learned all about HIV and AIDS, transmission, prevention, testing, teen pregnancy, STDs and drug abuse. I learned about peer pressure, good decision making skills, self esteem and leadership. The program also taught me how to prepare presentations and do public speaking....Now I'm not as shy and I can speak in front of an audience. Last year alone "Peers" conducted 67 presentations in the community.
>
> Programs like "Peers" are important in the fight to reduce risky behaviors among teens. I think that the Federal government could better serve the needs of adolescents by funding more groups and organizations to do creative education programs focused on different types of risky behavior. Also, the government could develop more comprehensive health care at existing clinics. I realize that I am only 15, but my experience says "adults will have to try some new methods or possibly lose many of today's youth."[90]

Community-wide coalitions of health providers, educational systems, youth serving agencies, parents, youth and others who are actively involved in the battle against adolescent HIV infection have been organized in a number of cities across the country. Coalitions have formed not only in large epicenters of the epidemic, but also in communities that have benefited from histories of coordination of public health and educational services.

Programs for Out-of-school Youth Also Require Broad Community Support

Many adolescents at highest risk of HIV infection have left school and require identification and vigorous outreach efforts. The Census Bureau estimated that 11% of all high school students -- at least 4,000,000 -- dropped out of school in 1988. In addition, more than a million youth are homeless, or run away from home every year. As many as 300,000 are long-term runaways who live on the streets, often supporting themselves by drug dealing and prostitution.[91] (See Chapter III for further discussion of the HIV-related needs of runaway and homeless youth and other out-of-school youth.)

Community-based agencies working with these high-risk populations are important settings for HIV prevention programming. A promising site for screening is the STD clinic, as youth engaged in high-risk behavior often contract sexually transmitted diseases other than HIV infection, and frequently seek medical help for such problems.[92]

Public facilities used primarily for other purposes can also house programs for out-of-school youth in high-risk situations. As a case in point, some city gymnasiums have started Midnight Basketball Leagues, a public/private partnership in which members of local business communities contribute financially to supply uniforms and equipment to teams of players who attend classes after games.

A witness at the "Risky Business" hearings, Gil Walker, Commissioner of Midnight Basketball in the Chicago Housing Authority, described his sports-linked program to the Committee:

> Midnight Basketball is a viable alternative to a lack of positive late night recreational options. The "hanging out" of young males...during the hours of 10 p.m. to 2 a.m. creates a climate which is conducive for negative activities, a notion confirmed by police statistics. In addition to utilizing basketball as an attractive, off-the-street activity, components have been added which are designed to encourage the participants to take charge of their own life, family and

destiny, i.e., Employment Development and Training, Life Planning and Group Motivation, Mentoring and Support Services Network.[93]

An independent university-based researcher in Chicago concluded that the Midnight Basketball League has been successful in motivating youth to avoid both high-risk behavior and encounters with the justice system, and has helped players complete GED diplomas and secure full-time employment. This is not surprising, as Midnight Basketball includes all of the strategies recently identified by researcher Joy Dryfoos as characteristic of programs that succeed in reducing risk: one-on-one individual attention from adults; involvement of parents; a focus on basic academics; and, community-wide, multi-agency approaches.[94]

Effective programs targeting extremely high-risk "street kids" include training in practical, realistic skills geared to their immediate needs, as it is easier to influence adolescents to modify behaviors than to discontinue them.[95] In other words, although discontinuing high-risk behavior altogether is to be encouraged, it must be recognized that cessation is not a realistic goal in many of these difficult cases. In addition to the usual prevention activities, program components needed for this target group may include drug or sexual abuse counseling, information about cleaning injection equipment,[96] and provision of basic economic assistance.[97]

Counseling may be a prerequisite for runaway youth to heed HIV prevention warnings. For example, since many runaways are sexually abused,[98] and sexual abuse is correlated with drug use,[99] counseling that addresses the emotional aftermath of sexual abuse may have the collateral advantage of reducing risk of HIV.

G. TEEN HIV PREVENTION FACES MAJOR BARRIERS

Teachers Need In-Service Training in HIV Prevention

According to a 1990 study by the General Accounting Office (GAO),[100] teachers should be better trained to impart HIV prevention information in culturally sensitive and developmentally appropriate ways. GAO also found that most teachers still require education in relevant technical matters such as the legal standing of adolescents and school personnel regarding testing, treatment, and anti-discrimination procedures.

Adequate in-service training deals with psychosocial topics relevant to HIV education.[101] Teachers often need to learn how to handle embarrassing or sensitive subjects.[102] They need sound advice about how to persuade students to change their own behavior and to exert positive peer pressure on members of their social groups.[103] Finally, teachers must learn how to help students make rational decisions when they are emotionally aroused, and how to teach assertiveness in intimate and social situations.[104] The mastery of these didactic skills should be included in evaluations of teacher training.

GAO found that, even when teaching HIV education courses, most teachers spend very few minutes on sensitive topics. This defeats preventive education goals because teens need practical suggestions, rehearsal, and same-sex as well as mixed discussions of what they have learned about avoiding risky behavior.[105]

Experts suggest that HIV education in schools should provide information about community resources, mechanisms of HIV transmission,[106] and clear descriptions of behaviors that put a person at risk. Teachers should not assume that adolescents are aware of risks entailed in unprotected homosexual and heterosexual sexual activity, in having multiple sexual partners, and in sharing needles and/or works during IV drug use, ear-piercing, etc.[107]

Other Barriers to School-Based Programming

Fear, Resistance and Apathy

Several factors make preventing HIV infection in adolescents very challenging. One commonly reported barrier is the fear felt by some adults of the results of frank discussion of sexual or risky behavior with adolescents.[108]

Sometimes this fear has led to open, active resistance to HIV prevention programming in schools. For example, parents have objected to particular items in questionnaires which they found overly explicit. While the objections were well meant, they blocked assessment of prevention needs.[109]

At other times, resistance has taken the form of public apathy or denial of the problem, a particularly serious obstacle in rural areas. A survey of HIV educators in rural America suggested strategies, including use of the highly respected county extension agents, to overcome denial and resistance.[110]

Resistance to plain talk has permeated the highest levels of research funding and national program policy.[111] A striking illustration is the current Administration's blockage of a large scale epidemiological study of adolescent sexual practices. AIDS researchers argue that the information is badly needed to update Kinsey's data from the 1940s because sexual mores and activity rates have changed so dramatically since that time, and because prevention resources are scarce and must be used in the most efficient manner.[112]

Gardner's testimony in the "Risky Business" hearings decried the fact that:

> Little is known about adolescent sexual practices or what they mean to youths. Development of effective, theory-based interventions requires support for basic research on adolescent behavior, and sexual behavior in particular.[113]

Even the CDC, the Federal public health agency responsible for HIV prevention in the public schools, avoids controversy around provision of explicit information by leaving decisions about which grades should offer self-protection information up to local communities. While such decisions are traditionally made at the local level, existing CDC guidelines could be interpreted to mean that it is safe to omit information about the protective value of condoms and spermicide from AIDS classes in middle schools. According to the Institute of Medicine, this omission could be dangerous because we know that some students in grades seven and eight are sexually active.

Witness Zedosky observed that collection of local risk data helps overcome denial of local problems:

> ...a Youth Risk Behavior Survey among our 9th through 12th grade students...gave us even more alarming data....23% reported that they already had as many as four sex partners. f our children are at risk.[114]

d number of additional strategies for overcoming thy and resistance to HIV prevention programs for en suggested.

SUGGESTIONS FROM
ATURE ON COMMUNITY SUPPORT
(*in no particular order*)

ents from the outset.

Organize broad-based coalitions with the support of diverse segments of the community to respond rapidly to opposition by articulating the importance of HIV education.

Translate AIDS programs into Spanish.

Make AIDS education part of a comprehensive, holistic, K-12 health education program included in the core curriculum.

Work slowly through trusted professionals in rural settings and anywhere resistance is anticipated.

Provide local physicians with educational material that answers student questions, perhaps videos made by people with AIDS.

Take field trips to agencies including health and family planning clinics, and drug abuse treatment centers.

Develop programs in conjunction with video-game arcades, movie theaters, and youth groups.

Work through adult mentoring programs.

Involve adolescents in community service like neighborhood watches and senior citizen escort programs to build self-esteem and promote integration into the community.

Recruit adults for telephone talk lines for teens.

Sources

Center for Population Options. Adolescents and HIV: A Community-Wide Responsibility. Washington, DC. 1989.

Kirby, D. (1990) Comprehensive school health and the larger community: Issues and a possible scenario. Journal of School Health, 60, 170-177.

McReynolds, V. (1990) What Works? HIV/AIDS Education in Rural America. Bellingham, Washington: National Rural and Small Schools Consortium.

Sabella, W. (1988) Introducing AIDS education in Connecticut schools. New England Journal of Medicine, 4, 335-346.

Wynn, et al. (1987) Communities and Adolescents: An Exploration of Reciprocal Supports. The Chapin Hall Center for Children, University of Chicago.

Health Care -- Including Promising School-Linked Health Services -- Not Readily Available to Youth

Adolescents' lack of access to health care presents another major barrier to providing HIV prevention services. As will be discussed in further detail in Chapter IV, medical care and psychological counseling are unavailable to large numbers of adolescents because of provider shortages, consent barriers, and lack of insurance coverage.

Testimony submitted to the Select Committee by the Center for Population Options discusses the role and increasing community acceptance of school-based clinics as a partial response to the access problem:

> A 1987 statement of the National PTA asserts that "school-linked health clinics are the only source of health care for many teens. They provide a wide variety of critical services such as immunizations, nutrition counseling, suicide prevention programs, drug and alcohol abuse prevention and treatment programs and general health assessments. By being on or near the school grounds, the health services are much more likely to be used."
>
> The school-based clinic movement is truly a grass-roots movement. Communities recognizing that lack of adequate health care services threatens the future of their adolescents and seeking workable solutions have given significant momentum to the movement. The number of identified SBCs increased four-fold between 1984 and 1989, from 31 to....At the present time...300 SBCs and school-linked clinics across the country.[115]

Some critics of school-based or school-linked health facilities are opposed to the perception that these facilities distribute contraceptive methods. However, by November 1991, only one in eight school-based or school-linked health facilities distributed condoms or had initiated plans to distribute them.

Respondents to an interview of HIV prevention programmers by Select Committee staff cited general health care, drug treatment and family planning services for teenagers as the areas of most critical service shortage. These shortages compound the threat of adolescent HIV infection, as discussed earlier in this chapter.

Insufficient Funding

Finally, insufficient resources have been allocated by states and the Federal Government to reach all teens in school with basic HIV and AIDS information.[116] The commitment to funding comprehensive prevention programs has simply not been made.[117]

Barriers to Serving Out-of-school Youth

Out-of-school youth are likely to face an additional set of barriers. While such problems can plague in-school youth as well, they are formidable obstacles to programming for adolescents who do not attend school. Barriers to serving these hard-to-reach youth include: (1) the isolation of these young people and their extreme lack of access to medical and social services; (2) their diminished trust of adults and authority figures; (3) the absence of other adult guidance and support; (4) their psychological problems, often including depression, anxiety, low self-esteem and suicidal ideation; (5) and, their behavioral problems, including high-risk sexual and drug activities.[118]

Some adults fear outreach to out-of-school youth as much as they do school-based programming, maintaining that information that reduces risk would encourage high-risk behavior. The fear has been expressed, for example, that teaching addicts to bleach needles after every intravenous injection would increase the frequency of drug use.[119]

Subtle community resistance has also been noted. It has been expressed by writing instructions for proper condom use at high reading levels, and placing condoms where teens must make themselves conspicuous by asking for them.[120]

Some communities have overcome their ambivalence and initiated "teenager friendly" condom distribution programs. Mayden described Maryland's "Three for Free" program at a Select Committee hearing:

> Condoms...and instructional material on correct condom use are provided in non-medical settings, where young men congregate. Typical sites include pool halls, barber shops, recreation centers, college campuses, restaurants and gas stations. In 1990, the Three for Free program with its 454 sites gave away 3,098,879 condoms in Maryland.[121]

There is no evidence that such programs increase sexual activity and thereby offset benefits.[122]

CHAPTER III

HARD-TO-REACH ADOLESCENTS AND YOUTH IN HIGH-RISK SITUATIONS REQUIRE TARGETED HIV PREVENTION AND SERVICES†

Preventing HIV and providing services to youth in high-risk situations present special demands. At particularly high risk of HIV are adolescents who engage in same-gender sexual behavior, those who have run away from home or are homeless, youth who are detained or incarcerated, those in foster care, and youth who use alcohol or other drugs. Other adolescents also require targeted interventions, including racial and ethnic minority youth, adolescents who have hemophilia, and those who have been sexually abused. Many of the unique HIV-related needs of each of these populations are detailed below.

A. HIV-RELATED NEEDS OF YOUTH ENGAGING IN SAME-GENDER SEXUAL BEHAVIOR

Experts suggest that same-gender sexual behavior is widespread among youth, but lack of reliable data has prevented accurate assessment of the prevalence of homosexual activity and risk-taking among youth who identify themselves as gay or lesbian. Male homosexual behavior is implicated in a large number of AIDS cases in teens and young adults, highlighting the urgent need for preventive interventions targeting this population. While formidable barriers impede effective HIV prevention efforts targeting youth engaging in same-gender sexual activity, existing models have shown marked success. In addition to the considerations addressed in Chapter II, programs for youth engaging in same-gender sexual behavior, particularly gay and lesbian youth, should also address self-esteem and support-seeking issues.

Same-Gender Sexual Behavior More Frequent Than Commonly Believed, New Data Needed

As found in Chapter I of this report, estimates of the extent of homosexual behavior among adolescents vary widely. In the

† Excerpted from CRS Report 102-1074

1940s and 1950s, Kinsey, et al. found that among adolescents, 28% of males and 17% of females reported at least one homosexual experience.[1] The Kinsey studies also found that nearly one out of ten adults reported either extensive or more than incidental homosexual experience, and nearly 40% reported *some* experience with same-gender sexual activity.[2]

Although outdated, the Kinsey studies still serve as a primary source of information on sexual behavior.[3] In fact, the Public Health Service uses Kinsey data to estimate HIV prevalence and forecast the AIDS epidemic.[4] The lack of more current data is particularly unfortunate because the methodology used for the Kinsey studies has been widely criticized, primarily due to sampling errors: The respondents were disproportionately drawn from the Midwest and college campuses, and the research did not use probability sampling.[5]

While the role of same-gender sexual contact in the sexual development of youth is unknown, significant numbers of adolescents who may not develop an exclusively homosexual identity or lifestyle do, nevertheless, experiment with same-gender sexual activity.[6]

The distinction between homosexual behavior and a homosexual orientation is important: HIV prevention efforts must address the risks of specific behaviors, regardless of the gender of the adolescent's partner. Adolescents who do not claim a homosexual identity, but are nevertheless engaging in risky homosexual behavior, may deny that risk.[7] Additionally, special effort must be made to reach adolescents who define themselves as gay or lesbian,[(a)] because these youth face formidable barriers to receiving appropriate HIV prevention messages.

(a) The 1989 U.S. Department of Health and Human Services report on youth suicide defines lesbian and gay male youth as young people who have a primary attraction to members of the same gender for sexual and intimate relationships.

Homosexual Activity is Significant Factor in AIDS Among Teens, Successful Prevention Programs for Gay Men Not Reaching Gay Youth

By the end of 1991, 60% of 13 to 24 year-old youth with AIDS reported male homosexual contact that could have exposed them to HIV.[8] The prevalence of HIV among gay youth is unknown. However, seroprevalence studies in 23 U.S. cities and 16 states found that HIV prevalence rates among adult gay men ranged from less than 10% to 70%, with most rates falling between 20%-50%.[9]

Since the early 1980s, gay-affiliated organizations have mobilized extensive HIV education and prevention campaigns. These efforts have produced some of the most profound modifications of personal health-related behaviors ever recorded.[10] Numerous cohort studies have shown that many gay men, particularly those living in urban areas, have significantly altered their high-risk behaviors, including decreasing the number of sexual partners and the frequency of unprotected anal intercourse.[11] These findings are supported by a gradual decline in the rate of increase of AIDS cases attributed to male homosexual contact, and a simultaneous reduction in the incidence of syphilis and gonorrhea among gay men compared with 1980 levels.[12]

However, as William Gardner testified before the Select Committee, the promising results of these studies cannot be generalized to all gay men or to gay adolescents.[13] In fact, the National Research Council found that young gay men engage in higher rates of risk taking than older gay men,[14] and other studies have found that gay youth are *less* likely than older gay men to perceive being at risk of HIV infection.[15]

In June 1991, the San Francisco Department of Public Health released "The Young Men's Survey," a study in which more than 250 young men ages 17-25 who self-identified as being gay/homosexual or bisexual, were interviewed.[16] Overall, one in eight interviewees was HIV seropositive and one in four was infected with Hepatitis B. Nearly one in ten reported having used intravenous drugs at least once, and 3% reported IV drug use in the six months prior to the survey. Moreover, HIV seroprevalence and the percent reporting risky sexual behavior were higher among teenage participants than among men in their early twenties. Table 1 summarizes data from the Young Men's Survey.

Table 1: Young Men's Survey - Prevalence of HIV, Hepatitis B, Unprotected Anal Sex and Oral Sex Among Young Gay and Bisexual Men, By Age[(b)]

AGES:	17-19 (n=21)	20-22 (n=93)	23-25 (n=144)
Seroprevalence of HIV	14.3	14.0	10.4
Seroprevalence of Hepatitis B	23.8	27.9	25.0
% Reporting Unprotected Anal Sex	42.9	24.7	29.9
% Reporting Unprotected Oral Sex	90.5	75.3	82.7

Findings from the Young Men's Study also show differences in seroprevalence and risk-taking behaviors when participants were compared by race and ethnicity. HIV and Hepatitis B seroprevalence and the frequency of unreported oral intercourse were highest among African-American participants, while HIV seroprevalence and the frequency of unprotected anal intercourse were lowest among Asian/Pacific Islander participants. Table 2 summarizes these data.

(b) San Francisco Department of Public Health, AIDS Office. "The Young Men's Survey: Principal Findings and Results - A Presentation to the San Francisco Health Commission." June 1991. Used with permission.

Table 2: Young Men's Survey - Prevalence of HIV, Hepatitis B, Unprotected Anal Sex and Oral Sex Among Young Gay and Bisexual Men, By Race/Ethnicity[(c)]

RACE/ETHNICITY	White (n=138)	Latino (n=49)	African-American (n=35)	Asian/Pac. Islander (n=33)
Seroprevalence of HIV	10.9	14.3	22.9	.0
Seroprevalence of Hepatitis B	24.6	22.4	40.0	24.2
% Reporting Unprotected Anal Intercourse	31.8	30.6	28.6	15.2
% Reporting Unprotected Oral Sex	81.8	77.5	85.7	75.8

Little Known About STDs and Risky Behaviors Among Youth Who Practice Same-Gender Sexual Behavior

Little is known about the prevalence of STDs or risky sexual and drug use practices among youth who practice same-gender sexual behavior.[17] Data are particularly lacking regarding the risk-taking behavior of lesbian girls, a group which is generally at very low risk of becoming pregnant or acquiring sexually transmitted diseases, including HIV.[18] One study used national AIDS case surveillance data to assess demographic characteristics and behavioral risk factors in adult and adolescent lesbians. This study found that between June 1980 and September 1989, of the 79 women with AIDS who reported sexual relations with only female partners, 95% were intravenous drug users. The authors also found that two instances of female-to-female transmission of HIV had been reported.[19]

In New York City, a study of HIV-related knowledge, attitudes, and behavior among runaway and gay male youth found that among the 60 primarily minority gay male youth interviewed, 77% were sexually active in the previous three months, including

(c) San Francisco Department of Public Health, AIDS Office. June 1991. op cit. Used with permission.

oral, anal, and vaginal intercourse and oral-anal contact. During this time, study participants reported a mean number of 4.1 partners and 22.8 sexual encounters. Almost one-half (44.1%) reported never using condoms and less than 15% reported consistent use of condoms. Bisexual activity was reported by nearly one-third (31.2%) of the gay male participants.[20]

High rates of risk-taking behavior have also been found among gay and bisexual youth from Minnesota. In one non-clinical study, gay and bisexual male youth reported a mean annual number of seven sexual partners. These youth reported that their partners were, on the average, seven years older, and that two-thirds of initial encounters occurred in bars or public meeting areas, with one-third of encounters being anonymous.[21] Because HIV and other STD rates are exceptionally high among adult gay men,[22] these data are extremely troubling. Nearly half of the youth interviewed for this study had a past history of sexually transmitted diseases, and the majority met professionally recognized criteria for substance abuse.[23]

Despite significant gaps in knowledge about the behaviors of youth engaging in same-gender sexual behavior, numerous studies show that this population has an urgent need for improved HIV prevention interventions.[24]

Preventing HIV Among Youth Engaging in Homosexual Behavior Faces Significant Barriers

Stress to Conform Can Lead to Denial of Risk Taking

The process of acquiring a homosexual identity generally begins in early childhood and continues throughout adulthood.[25] During early adolescence, youth first experience heterosexual and homosexual attractions and fantasies.[26] Youth who feel an attraction to persons of the same gender often feel uncomfortable identifying with the stereotypes of gay and lesbian people that are prevalent in their environment and fear being associated with a group that is widely stigmatized by society.[27] As noted by the American Academy of Pediatrics:

> The social consequences of homosexual orientation in an adolescent include potential difficulties in peer group acceptance, family rejection, school and institutional harassment, limited employment opportunities, legal difficulties, and social isolation. Although homosexual orientation does not appear to predispose to mental illness, the social consequences of this life-style in a teenager may create serious emotional problems.[28]

The social stigma of homosexuality specifically impedes a young gay or lesbian's learning about AIDS.[29] Confronting immense pressure by their peers to conform, many young adolescents who practice same-gender sexual behavior do not identify themselves as gay, lesbian, or bisexual.[30] When homosexually active male youth deny their homosexual feelings, they may also deny the risks associated with their behavior.[31]

Additionally, youth who are attracted to persons of the same gender often seek heterosexual partners in order to confirm, hide, or attempt to "change" their emerging sexual identity.[32] In 1990, the General Accounting Office (GAO) found that this experimentation may serve as a possible link between homosexual and heterosexual youth in the transmission of HIV.[33] GAO also found that social pressures to engage in heterosexual relationships place lesbian youth, who would normally be less likely to engage in high-risk sexual behaviors, at increased risk of infection.[34]

Youth who eventually accept a homosexual orientation typically pass through stages of "coming out," during which they develop self-esteem, and the socialization skills needed to maintain friendships and intimate relationships.[35] During this developmental process, these youth continuously assess whether to disclose their identity and risk harassment or discrimination.[36] Their isolation complicates delivery of services, including risk reduction programs, because many gay and lesbian youth fear their sexual orientation will be discovered if they try to obtain needed help.[37]

Gay and Lesbian Youth Often Confront Rejection and Violence in Settings That Traditionally Provide HIV Prevention Services

Most adolescents cope successfully with the stress of these conflicting feelings about their sexual orientation. However, youth who feel more certain about their gay or lesbian identity face significant and sometimes overwhelming challenges to developing healthy self-esteem and relationships.[38] Most often, they are forced to make the difficult choice between either hiding their identity or confronting rejection, prejudice, and violence by friends, family, and other important adults.

As described earlier, school settings have the potential to reach nearly 45 million youth with HIV prevention curricula. However, as Gardner testified before the Select Committee, gay youth are difficult to reach through traditional school or public health interventions.[39] Gay and lesbian students often face ridicule from teachers, fellow students, and administrators who fail to punish verbal attacks on them.[40] A 1984 survey of over 2,000 gay and lesbian adults found that 45% of gay males and almost 20% of lesbians had experienced verbal or physical assault in secondary school.[41] School-based HIV prevention efforts that fail to provide positive support to gay and lesbian youth are less likely to have a significant impact on this population.[42]

Parents of gay and lesbian youth may also be unable or unwilling to reinforce HIV prevention messages. In fact, violence and harassment in school are often reinforced at home. A study by the Hetrick-Martin Institute, which serves gay and lesbian youth in New York City, found that of 500 young people seeking assistance in 1988, 40% reported having experienced violent physical assaults by family, peers, and strangers. Sixty-one percent of gay-related violence against these youth was perpetrated by family members.[43]

Many Gay and Lesbian Youth Respond Negatively to Stress with Increased Risk Taking

In response to such extreme pressures, many young lesbian and gay people suffer from poor self-esteem, feelings of isolation, and chronic depression.[44] Others rely on ultimately self-destructive coping behaviors and find themselves in situations that increase their risk of acquiring HIV. As Andy Humm, an educator with the Hetrick-Martin Institute noted, "The most important thing for a gay kid is to feel he has a future...when you feel you're alone in the world, that leads you to a lot of dangerous behaviors."[45]

While national studies have not been conducted, small scale studies indicate that gay and lesbian youth are at increased risk of alcohol and other drug abuse and school failure.[46] These indicators subsequently reduce the likelihood that HIV prevention messages will be heard or heeded.[47]

Rejected by friends and family, some gay and lesbian youth turn to life in the streets for emotional and financial support.[48] An estimated 25% of all youth living on the streets are gay, lesbian, bisexual, or transsexual.[49] (See "HIV-Related Needs of Runaway and Homeless Youth" in this chapter for further analysis of the risks associated with this high-risk situation.)

Suicide is the third leading cause of death among males and females ages 15-24, accounting for 8% of deaths among women and 15% of deaths among men in this age group in 1988.[50] In 1989, the U.S. Department of Health and Human Services (DHHS) found that gay and lesbian youth are two to three times more likely to attempt suicide than their peers, comprising up to 30% of completed youth suicides annually.[51]

A more recent study supports the DHHS findings. A 1991 study found that among nearly 140 males from Minnesota and Washington State who identified themselves as gay or bisexual, 30% reported at least one suicide attempt at a mean age of 15.5 years. Nearly one-half of those who had attempted suicide also reported other attempts to take their lives. One-third of first attempts occurred in the same year that the participants identified their sexual orientation. Eighty-five percent of attempters also reported illicit drug use, and 22% had undergone chemical dependency treatment.[52]

Social and Resource Barriers to Reaching Youth Who Practice Same-Gender Sexual Behavior Prevail

As described in Chapter II, successful HIV prevention programs must be culturally sensitive and instill precise information, a sense of vulnerability and self-efficacy, and skills.

These "protect yourself" messages should be reinforced by parents, schools, peers, churches and other community organizations. With respect to efforts aimed at gay adolescents:

> The effectiveness of AIDS prevention efforts for gay adolescents is enhanced by other programs to foster self-esteem, positive identity, and community. In the absence of family and peer support, adult role models, employment, shelter, and food, the power of education to affect behavioral changes rapidly dissipates.[53]

As has been mentioned previously, many HIV prevention programs, particularly those offered in schools, do not address the needs specific to lesbian and gay youth.[54] In 1989, the National Education Association took an important step in addressing this problem, by adopting a resolution which stated:

> All persons, regardless of sexual orientation, should be afforded equal opportunity within the public education system. The Association further believes that every school district should provide counseling for students who are struggling with their sexual/gender orientation.[55]

However, this commitment is not widespread among service providers from the juvenile justice, child welfare, and health care services who have historically neither identified nor addressed the special needs of this population.[56] Moreover, most schools and youth-serving agencies do not have policies, programming, or staff training to help these youth develop strong self-esteem and a sense of self-efficacy to prevent or reduce HIV-related risk-taking behaviors.[57]

Other political barriers include a lack of Federal resources dedicated to HIV prevention serving gay and lesbian youth. This is particularly disturbing, given the high proportion of AIDS cases among youth that are linked to homosexual behavior, and data that indicate that many of these youth engage in sexual and drug use behaviors that put them at risk of HIV.[58] Additionally, Federal restrictions on explicit information about safer sex practices for these youth make it difficult to provide the information they need to protect themselves and their partners from HIV.[59]

Several Model Programs Making Inroads to Prevent HIV Among Gay and Bisexual Male Youth

Several model programs providing HIV prevention services to gay male youth exist and are noteworthy because they have overcome many of the barriers addressed above.

One model HIV prevention program, at the HIV Center for Clinical and Behavioral Studies at Columbia University, has produced significant reductions in risky behavior among nearly 150 predominantly Hispanic (51%) and African-American (31%) gay males ages 14-19. This program provides intensive HIV prevention services, including individual risk assessment and counseling, coping skills training sessions, and facilitated access to comprehensive medical and social services. After one year, 57% of program participants reported increased condom use. An additional 18% of participants reported decreases in unprotected sex and then relapsed. Improvements were greater for African-American youths than for Hispanic youths who engaged in significantly fewer risk acts initially, but made fewer behavior changes over time.[60]

A second model program targeting gay male youth is conducted by the Department of Pediatrics at the University of Minnesota. The Youth and AIDS Project (YAP) provides comprehensive outreach, risk reduction counseling, peer education, case management, referral for medical and psychosocial services, and longitudinal follow-up to youth who self-identify as gay or bisexual. Program participants include 140 males ages 14-21, more than half of whom grew up in non-urban areas, principally in Minnesota.[61]

Initial data from YAP indicate that 75% engaged in unprotected anal intercourse and/or needle sharing, nearly one-fifth (18%) were chemically dependent, and the same number (18%) of participants reported a history of sexually transmitted diseases. Additionally, 83% of participants did not know that HIV can be transmitted through oral sex, 16% denied any risk for HIV, and 12% were unaware of the HIV antibody test.[62]

After participating in YAP for three months, the young men

reported a sharp increase in consistent use of condoms during anal intercourse (from 44% to 73%), and were significantly less likely to report oral sex and symptoms of dysfunctional substance abuse.[63] Perceived personal vulnerability to HIV increased by 15% among YAP participants and denial of any personal risk for HIV decreased from 16% to 6%. Additionally, regular use of alcohol in sexual situations diminished from 17% to 4%, involvement in prostitution decreased from 8% to 0%, and consistent use of condoms with new partners more than doubled from 30% to 65%.[64]

B. HIV-RELATED NEEDS OF HOMELESS AND RUNAWAY YOUTH

Estimates of the Number of Homeless and Runaway Youth Vary, But Too Many Teens Forced to Survive on the Streets

Adolescents live on the streets for a variety of reasons. Many children run away from home each year, while others are literally "thrown away" or abandoned by their families. The Office of Juvenile Justice and Delinquency Prevention (OJJDP) estimates that in 1988, 450,700 youth ran away from their homes or juvenile institutions across the United States. Of this group, nearly 130,000 youth were without a secure and familiar place to stay. Additionally, OJJDP estimates that in 1988 more than 127,000 children were thrown away or abandoned by parents or guardians, and more than 59,000 youth did not have a secure and familiar place to stay during some portion of the time they spent away from their homes.[65]

Other studies indicate higher estimates of homeless and runaway youth. The National Network on Youth and Runaway Services estimates that the number of youth permanently living on the streets ranges from 100,000 to 300,000, with as many as 1,300,000 to 2,000,000 running away from home each year.[66] Community and youth shelter surveys suggest that each year between 1,000,000 - 1,300,000 adolescents live on the streets or receive services from emergency shelters. A large portion of these adolescents are runaways.[67] Another study estimates that the actual number of adolescents on the streets and in emergency shelters may be closer to 500,000.[68]

Although estimates on the number of runaway and homeless youth vary, it is clear that each year significant numbers of youth are forced to survive living on the streets.

Rate of HIV Infection Among Runaway and Homeless Youth Unknown, Rates High Among Youth in Shelters

The extent of HIV infection among runaway and homeless adolescents is unknown. However, several youth shelters have collected HIV seroprevalence data from youth whom they serve. These studies indicate a wide range of infection rates.

One study of nearly 2,700 youth who received services at Covenant House in New York City between October 1987 and 1989 found that more than 5% were infected with HIV. Data from this study indicate that the longer an adolescent was homeless, the more likely he or she was to be infected with HIV -- the average rate of HIV infection for youth age 20 was 8.6%.[69] Another anonymous seroprevalence study conducted at a New York health clinic for runaway youth noted that 7% of the youth tested were infected with HIV.[70]

Additionally, a 1991 survey conducted by the Inspector General of the DHHS found that HIV seroprevalence varies by city. Among youth served by a clinical program in a large east coast city, three of every ten were infected with HIV, compared with three of every 100 tested among youth served by a shelter in a large southern city.[71]

Successful HIV Prevention Among Homeless and Runaway Youth Faces Formidable Barriers

Numerous barriers impede successful HIV prevention for runaway and homeless youth. These include: Stressful situations encountered by living on the street; lack of education, job skills, medical care, and social services; increased drug and alcohol use; and unrealistic stereotypes about these youth. As noted by Rotheram-Borus:

> The lack of supportive resources and the existence of multiple problem behaviors and emotional distress must be considered

in the design, implementation, and evaluation of HIV-related services for homeless youths. As one adolescent in a shelter expressed the problem: "Why should I care about dying ten years from now when I do not know where I will sleep and how I will get food tomorrow." The risk of HIV infection can only be addressed in the context of the youths' lives.[72]

Runaway and Homeless Youth Encounter Stress at Home and on the Streets

The failure to have a supportive and "functional" family may be the single largest factor associated with adolescent homelessness.[73] Lack of support ranges from strained interpersonal relationships to parental substance abuse, which may lead to neglect, and physical, emotional, and sexual abuse. The trauma of these problems can affect how runaway and homeless youth cope with high-risk situations.

A 1989 GAO study of the characteristics of youth served by shelters provides additional evidence of the prevalence of family problems among runaway and homeless youth. GAO interviewed youth as well as experts in the field, and found that almost one-half of the youth had emotional conflicts with their parents, more than one in four suffered parental neglect, more than one in four suffered from prior physical or sexual abuse, almost one in five had parents who abused drugs or alcohol, more than one in five thought that their parents were too strict, and approximately one in ten observed domestic violence within their homes.[74]

The rate of sexual abuse prior to street life among homeless and runaway youth may be higher than the GAO estimates. In 1988, Maureen Gammon, a community health outreach worker at the Larkin Street Youth Center in San Francisco, estimated that of the 75 homeless teenagers seen at the center during the average week, over 60% were sexually abused prior to leaving home.[75]

A 1991 study of 50 homeless adolescents by the Stanford Center for the Study of Families, Children and Youth found that more than half reported having been physically abused, and nearly four in ten reported having been sexually abused by family members. More than half of these youth reported parental alcoholism, and almost four in ten reported drug abuse by their parents. The connection between abuse within the home and homelessness was described by one youth interviewed for the Stanford study: "I would rather be homeless. It is cold and miserable on the streets, but it is better than being beaten up by parents who don't care."[76]

Sexual abuse within the home not only serves as a precipitating factor in running away, but it may also be linked to high-risk behavior of runaway and homeless youth including increased sexual activity.[77] (See "Considerations for Serving Youth Who Have Been Sexually Abused" in this chapter for further discussion of these issues.)

As discussed in the previous section of this report, many gay and lesbian youth are rejected by their families and forced to leave home. According to a recent report from the Technical Assistance Center of the Child and Adolescent Service System Program (CASSP), shelters report an "increase in the number of gay and lesbian youth who have been rejected by their families because of their sexual preference."[78] The Seattle Department of Human Resources reports approximately 40% of runaway and homeless youth are gay.[79] Andrew Humm, Director of Education at the Hetrick-Martin Institute estimates that as many as one half of youth on the streets of New York are gay or lesbian.[80]

Emotionally and physically abused youth who live on the streets find themselves in a situation in which any individual would have difficulty coping. As noted by the Center for Population Options:

> Undereducated, often abused, and lacking a family support system that provides needed direction, homeless and runaway youth are forced to make painful decisions. Their lack of marketable skills and their status as minors leave them with few legitimate alternatives to illegal activities. Many become involved in prostitution, pornography, and the illegal drug trade to pay for food or a place to stay.[81]

Prostitution, "Survival Sex," Rape, High Rates of Pregnancy and Alcohol and Other Drug Use Put Homeless and Runaway Youth at Increased Risk of HIV

High-risk behaviors practiced by runaway and homeless youth are generally the same ones found among the general adolescent population at large: unprotected sex; sex with multiple partners; and the use of alcohol and other illicit drugs. Like non-homeless youth, runaway and homeless youth are subject to rape.

In order to survive on the streets, runaway and homeless youth may resort to prostitution or "survival sex" (the exchange of sex for food, shelter, money, or drugs), although estimates of these behaviors in runaway and homeless youth vary from 5% to 80%.[82]

Survival sex by itself constitutes high-risk behavior. Yet, the risk involved with survival sex can be enhanced by pressures placed on runaway and homeless youth. Anecdotal evidence suggests that youth engaged in prostitution may earn more money from "tricks" or "johns" if they do not use a condom during intercourse or oral sex. According to Jay Coburn, Director of the Safe Choices Project of the National Network of Runaway and Youth Services, "The adults who sexually assault or exploit these teenagers are rarely interested in risk reduction; they pay and/or coerce youth to forego condom use."[83] In 1988, Washington, D.C. customers offered prostitutes $50 to $500 to have intercourse without a condom.[84] As noted by Athey, Chief of the Public Health Social Work Division within the Maternal and Child Health Bureau of DHHS, "Clearly, to the extent that survival sex involves multiple partners and is unprotected, HIV risk is increased."[85]

One 1988 study compared the health status of 765 runaway and non-runaway youth who were served by Children's Hospital of Los Angeles and the Los Angeles Free Clinic. More than one in four runaway youth reported that they engaged in survival sex compared with fewer than one in ten non-runaway youth. Runaway youth were four times more likely to report sexual abuse, eight times more likely to report physical abuse, and three times more likely to report being raped than were non-runaway youth. In addition, more than half of the runaway youth had dropped out of high school compared with one in ten non-runaway youth. As outlined in Table 3, runaway youth used alcohol and other drugs more frequently than the non-runaway population. [86]

Table 3: Percent of Runaway and Homeless Youth Reporting Alcohol and Other Drug Use Compared with Non-Runaway Youth[(d)]

Drugs	Runaways (N=110)	Non-Runaways (N=655)
IV Drug Use	34.5%	3.7%
Hallucinogens	22.7%	2.4%
Stimulants	36.4%	7.0%
Inhalants	6.4%	2.4%
Narcotics	13.6%	3.4%
Alcohol	54.5%	49.9%
Cigarettes	42.7%	34.2%
Drug Problem	7.3%	1.1%
Marijuana	44.5%	28.7%
No Drug Use	16.4%	33.0%

GAO also found that approximately 20% of homeless and runaway youth reported using drugs and alcohol.[87]

Rates of consistent condom use among homeless and runaway youth vary. Another study found that prior to HIV prevention sessions only one-fourth of runaway youth reported consistent condom use during the previous 3 months; and 80% reported never having used condoms.[88]

One proxy of failure to use contraceptives, including latex condoms, is pregnancy: The pregnancy rate among homeless adolescents is higher than among non-homeless youth. A 1989 study of females ages 16-19 in 19 cities found that more than one

(d) Yates, G.L., et al. July 1988. op cit.

in three homeless females was pregnant, compared with approximately one in ten females who were not homeless.[89] Although this study found that sexually transmitted diseases were three times as frequent among homeless females, other studies have found an equal prevalence of STDs among homeless and non-homeless females.[90]

Rape is a hazard for all runaway and homeless youth, especially females. According to Athey:

> ...the rate of sexual assault on homeless women is reported to be approximately 20 times the rate among women in general. Nationally, 50% of all rape victims are less than 18 years old. Since homeless girls have the double risk factors of youth and homelessness, it can be assumed that rape is a common experience for them.[91]

One New York City shelter reported that 25% of adolescent females experienced rape sometime during their lives.[92] Rape of male runaway and homeless youth is also not uncommon.[93]

Runaway and Homeless Youth Find Doors To Traditional Sources of Prevention Messages and Treatment Closed, Need for Parental Consent Also Impedes Access to Care

Although youth living on the streets are reported to have a general knowledge about HIV infection[94], they often do not participate in traditional educational activities which could give them a more comprehensive understanding of HIV infection and skills for reducing high-risk behavior. According to Coburn:

> Youth at highest risk for HIV infection face the same developmental challenges as other youth....As far as HIV, they are often isolated from the institutions that are typically expected to carry prevention messages -- schools, families, and health services.[95]

In its 1991 Adolescent Health report, OTA found that many HIV prevention programs are family- or school-based and not geared toward runaway and homeless youth. As detailed in Chapter II, community-based programs, such as teen street theater, "rap" and poster contests, distribution of printed materials, STD and AIDS hotlines, individual and group counseling, media campaigns, condom distribution and needle exchange and bleach programs exist, but very few have been evaluated for effectiveness.[96] It is also unclear to what extent the community programs consider and serve the needs of runaway and homeless youth.[97]

Because they live on the streets, runaway and homeless youth fail to receive prevention messages through the mail and television.[98] Other resources necessary for preventing HIV may also be unavailable to runaway and homeless youth. For example, although they may know that cleaning needles and syringes in a chlorine solution will sterilize them, runaway and homeless youth often lack access to bleach or a private place where they can clean these items.[99]

Moreover, various studies have found that runaway and homeless youth often fail to attend school.[100] One study found that more than seven in ten boys and almost five in ten girls who live on the streets either drop out or are expelled from school.[101]

Many health care institutions also provide HIV prevention materials, including condoms, but these services are rarely accessible to runaway and homeless youth. The Office of the Inspector General found that due to lack of funds or the inability to meet eligibility requirements, many homeless and runaway youth are unable to gain access to health care and social services.[102] Also, traditional health care institutions often reject runaway and homeless youth, "considering them to be either a poor risk or to carry problems too complex to handle."[103]

The 1991 Inspector General study highlighted various problems that inhibit HIV prevention, testing, and treatment efforts on behalf of runaway and homeless youth. Even when services are apparently available to youth in the community, requirements such as money, parental consent and age restrictions, fragmentation of funding sources, and different ideological approaches "weaken service delivery for runaway and homeless youth with or at risk of HIV infection."[104] As discussed elsewhere in this report, although early detection of HIV can reduce the spread of the infection, shelter staff remain reluctant to test youth at risk of infection due to the lack of proper counseling and available follow-up services.

Many studies have also found that Federal and state policies impede the participation of runaway and homeless youths' participation in AIDS clinical trials, particularly requirements for parental consent.[105]

Stereotypes About Homeless and Runaway Youth Thwart Prevention Efforts and Treatment

It is important to note that while many runaway and homeless youth are faced with difficult and dangerous situations, health care providers and policymakers often have inaccurate beliefs about the lives of these youth. Recently, in testimony before the Select Committee on Children, Youth, and Families, Mary Jane Rotheram-Borus observed that:

> The stereotypes do not focus on the fact that 25% of these youths are sexually abstinent, or the fact that female runaways typically have been sexually involved with only one partner in the past three months, with males typically involved with 2-4 partners in the same time period, and that their condom use is similar to that of adolescents in general.[106]

GAO confirms this observation, finding that media portrayals of runaway and homeless youth which highlight drug abuse or prostitution are often exaggerated. According to GAO, "The majority of homeless youth were not reported to have such problems (i.e., drug abuse and prostitution). Approximately one in five was reported as having a drug or alcohol problem, while approximately one in seven females had to deal with pregnancy or venereal disease."[107]

The stereotype that homeless and runaway youth are beyond help inhibits many prevention and health care providers from serving runaway and homeless youth. Rotheram-Borus criticizes the widely held opinion of one reviewer for the Journal of the American Medical Association, who wrote that the "bleak and hopeless future" of runaway and homeless youth and concludes that "the problem is so huge, so inevitable; nothing can be done."[108]

Model HIV Prevention Programs for Runaway and Homeless Youth Are Intensive, Combine Skills Development with Access to Comprehensive Health Care Services

When the special needs of runaway and homeless youth are addressed in long-term intervention sessions, risk-taking behavior of runaway and homeless youth decreases. A 1991 study examined the high-risk behavior of 145 runaways at residential shelters and evaluated the impact of comprehensive intervention (up to 30 sessions) on their behavior. Sessions included discussions of general knowledge of HIV/AIDS, coping skills, access to resources and individual counseling to reduce barriers to safer sex. Youth who received the comprehensive intervention reported an increase in condom use and a decrease in high-risk behavior.[109]

In testimony before the Select Committee, the program's Director, Rotheram-Borus compared her program with teenage pregnancy, substance abuse, and smoking prevention efforts that have produced behavior change:

> These programs share several characteristics: a) Interventions are provided in the context of making available comprehensive health care services and other community resources; b) they build on participants' strengths rather than merely targeting deficits; c) they engage participants in active rehearsal of the targeted health-enhancing behaviors; d) social support from peers in the environment reinforces learning; and the interventions are intensive, providing, for example, 15 or more sessions instead of merely 2-3 hours of educational interventions.[110]

Prior to entering the shelters, fewer than one in four runaways reported consistent condom use in the last three months, and among sexually active youth, almost one in four reported engaging in high-risk sexual behavior, defined by the number of partners and sexual encounters, as well as condom use. After six months of intervention, more than six in ten youth reported consistent condom use. <u>No</u> youth reported participating in high-risk behaviors, defined as infrequent condom use (condom use during 0-49% of sexual encounters) combined with ten or more sexual encounters and/or with three or more sexual partners.[111]

The "Safe Choices" project sponsored by the National Network of Runaway and Youth Services provides HIV prevention training to community-based agencies that serve youth in high-risk situations, including homeless and runaway youth. Components of the Safe Choices project include train-the-trainer workshops, technical assistance to community-based organizations regarding model program components, policy development, funding sources, and new materials, and various hotlines and publications which include a model training manual.[112]

Experts Recommend Comprehensive HIV Prevention and Services for Runaway and Homeless Youth

In 1991, the American Medical Association identified the following needs and recommendations regarding the health care of runaway and homeless adolescents:

- Funding should be provided by an appropriate government agency for a national study that would provide accurate, timely, and reliable data on homeless adolescents;
- Conduct a pilot study of the health care needs of homeless youth in order to provide physicians with solid baseline data on this issue;
- Establish a protocol to be used in the evaluation and treatment of homeless youth;
- Disseminate information on the lack of treatment facilities and health care providers for treating homeless youth;
- Encourage state medical societies to determine the extent of treatment possible under state law, to inform physicians of the laws and regulations affecting the treatment of minors, and to form linkages with statewide youth advocacy groups to develop protocols for the treatment of troubled youth; and,

- Encourage local medical societies to develop and publicize lists of local and regional resources that can assist homeless adolescents, to provide this information to local physicians, and to establish links with providers of youth services to improve knowledge of the needs and limitations of these youth and physicians who provide care.[113]

In addition, a 1991 literature review of homeless youth and HIV infection included several recommendations about serving homeless and runaway youth. The authors found that standard one- or two-day "AIDS 101" sessions have little effect on the behavior of runaway and homeless youth. They also recommended providing comprehensive care, including case management, to HIV-infected adolescents specifically targeted to homeless youth, and proposed increased Federal and state funding of HIV prevention programs in temporary shelters, foster care and group home settings, and other social service agencies.[114]

Strategies have been outlined to improve service delivery to runaway and homeless youth who are infected with HIV. These include a holistic and comprehensive approach to service delivery provided by multi-agency coordinated care and "wrap-around" services. Multi-agency coordinated care would address the problems caused by incomplete and fragmented care by providing a comprehensive system of care which uses "interagency committees, multi-disciplinary teams, and 'blended funding', accompanied by case management." Wrap-around services would assure that if a particular youth's needs are not being met by the system, a program will be designed to meet the specific needs of that youth.[115]

C. HIV-RELATED NEEDS OF INCARCERATED AND DETAINED YOUTH

Although studies of limited samples indicate that large percentages of youth who reside in corrections facilities have engaged in behavior that puts them at risk of HIV infection, no regular or periodic assessment of HIV infection or of high-risk behavior is conducted in these settings. Little is known about either the quality or the availability of health care, health education, or disease prevention services for youth in custody.[116] As noted by the National Commission on AIDS, "For the most part, juvenile facilities continue to suffer from extreme inattention. Information regarding access and quality of health care must be obtained and made available."[117] However, the limited information that is available indicates that the need for increased HIV prevention, drug treatment, and medical services for youth in correctional facilities cannot be overstated.

Prevalence of HIV Among Adult Inmates is Staggering, Rates Among Juveniles in Custody Unknown

Since 1985, the National Institute of Justice (NIJ) has reported the number of AIDS cases confirmed among adult inmates in U.S. Federal, state, and selected large city/county correctional facilities. By the end of November 1989, this number had reached 5,411 representing a 72% increase over the previous year.[118] In fact, for the first time since NIJ has sponsored this survey, the percent increase in cumulative correctional AIDS cases exceeded the increase in AIDS cases reported in the U.S. population at large, which had a 50% increase over the previous year. AIDS has become the leading cause of death in several correctional systems.[119] Additionally, the prevalence of HIV among nearly 11,000 consecutive entrants to ten correctional systems in 1988-1989 ranged from 2.1% to 7.6% for men and 2.5% to 14.7% among women.[120]

The rate of HIV infection and AIDS among youth in correctional facilities is unknown. A seroprevalence study of nearly 1,900 youth admitted to two Los Angeles County juvenile facilities during a seven-month period in 1987 found that 0.16% of youth were infected with HIV.[121] In a 1989 survey of 1,400 public and private juvenile facilities, 14 cases of AIDS were confirmed and responding institutions reported two AIDS-related deaths. These numbers represent a minimum estimate, because not all facilities were surveyed, and less than one-third of those contacted actually responded.[122]

Several smaller studies indicate that, by virtue of their participation in risky sexual and drug use behaviors, and their limited access to medical, social, and other preventative services, detained and incarcerated youth are at increased risk of HIV infection.

Numbers of Incarcerated and Detained Youth Rose Dramatically During the 1980s

As shown in Table 4, 95,621 youth were held in public and private juvenile facilities and adult jails during a one-day census of these facilities during 1989.[(e)]

Table 4. Juveniles Held in Public and Private Facilities and Adult Jails During a One-Day Census in 1989[(f)]

	Males	Females	Total
Public Juvenile Facilities	49,443	6,680	56,123
Private Juvenile Facilities	26,602	11,220	37,822
Adult Jails	1,564	112	1,676
Total	**77,609**	**18,012**	**95,621**

The number of juveniles in custody has increased dramatically during the past decade. Between 1979 and 1989, the number of youth held in juvenile facilities (public and private)

(e) The numbers presented in this section reflect a one-day count; many more youth go through these facilities during the course of the year.

In 1988, there were 619,181 admissions to public juvenile facilities, 141,463 to private juvenile facilities, and 65,263 juveniles were admitted to adult jails. The number of admissions may count an individual more than once if he or she was transferred between facilities or entered the system more than once during the year. (U.S. Department of Justice. Office of Juvenile Justice and Delinquency Prevention [OJJDP]. Juveniles Taken Into Custody: Fiscal Year 1990 Report. National Council on Crime and Delinquency, San Francisco, CA. September 1991).

(f) OJJDP. September 1991. op cit.

NOTE: Few data exist regarding the nearly 1,700 juveniles held in adult jails. The remainder of this section will focus on youth held in juvenile facilities.

increased by 31%.[123] By 1989, the number of youth held in public juvenile facilities reached its highest number since the Department of Justice conducted the first Children in Custody census in 1971.[(g)]

Moreover, the juvenile custody rates in public facilities per 100,000 population increased by 19% from 1985 to 1989, reflecting both an increase in the number of detained and incarcerated youth and a decrease in the absolute numbers of U.S. youth ages 10-19.[124]

As shown in Table 5, 70% of juveniles in public and private facilities during a one-day census in 1989 were held for delinquent offenses, acts that would be crimes if committed by adults. One in ten juveniles was held for status offenses, such as truancy or running away, and 20% were detained or committed for reasons not involving offenses, such as abuse or neglect by parents.

(g) Children in Custody is a biennial survey published by the Office of Juvenile Justice and Delinquency Prevention that provides data regarding children in public juvenile detention, correctional, and shelter facilities.

Table 5: Selected Demographic Characteristics of Juveniles Held in Public and Private Facilities During a One-Day Census in 1989[(h)]

	Public Facilities	(%)	Private Facilities	(%)	Total Facilities	(%)
ALL JUVENILES	56,123	(60%)	37,822	(40%)	93,945	(100%)
GENDER						
Males	49,443	(88%)	26,602	(70%)	76,045	(81%)
Females	6,680	(12%)	11,220	(30%)	17,900	(19%)
RACE/ETHNICITY						
White	22,201	(40%)	22,807	(60%)	45,008	(48%)
Black	23,836	(42%)	10,883	(29%)	34,719	(37%)
Hispanic	8,671	(16%)	3,082	(8%)	11,753	(13%)
Other	1,415	(2%)	1,050	(3%)	2,465	(2%)
AGE AT CENSUS						
9 and under	45	(*)	718	(2%)	763	(1%)
10-13 years	3,276	(6%)	5,917	(16%)	9,193	(10%)
14-17 years	44,894	(80%)	29,688	(78%)	74,582	(79%)
18-21 years	7,908	(14%)	1,499	(4%)	9,407	(10%)
ADJUDICATION STATUS						
Detained	17,612	(31%)	2,593	(7%)	20,205	(21%)
Committed	38,209	(68%)	28,269	(75%)	66,478	(71%)
Voluntary	302	(1%)	6,960	(18%)	7,262	(8%)
REASONS FOR ADMISSION/CUSTODY						
Delinquent Acts	53,037	(95%)	13,095	(35%)	66,132	(70%)
Status Offenders	2,245	(4%)	6,853	(18%)	9,098	(10%)
Non-Offenders	841	(1%)	17,874	(47%)	18,715	(20%)

* Denotes less than 0.5%.

(h) OJJDP. September 1991. op cit; Barbara Allen-Hagen Research and Program Development Division, OJJDP, Personal Communication, February, 1992.

Table 6 summarizes data provided in the Children in Custody, 1989 report regarding youth held in public juvenile facilities during a one-day census in 1989.

Table 6: Profile of Selected Characteristics of Youth in Public Juvenile Facilities During a One-Day Census, 1989[i]

More than nine out of ten (95%) of all juveniles in public facilities were held for delinquent offenses, acts that would be crimes if committed by adults. Four percent were held for status offenses such as truancy or running away. Just over 1% were detained or committed because they were abused, neglected, or dependent youth, were held for reasons not involving juvenile offenses, or were admitted on a voluntary basis.

The number of juveniles held for alcohol or drug offenses increased by nearly 150% between 1985 and 1989. Nearly 11% of all juveniles in public facilities in 1989 were held for drug-related offenses. Of these, almost one-half (49%) were held for distribution of drugs.

Males account for 88% of juveniles in public custody. The percent of females in public juvenile facilities decreased by 8% between 1987 and 1989.

Four out of five juveniles in correctional facilities are between the ages of 14 and 17 years. However, between 1987 and 1989, the percent of younger children (ages 10-13 years) and older youth (ages 18 and older) increased by 17% and 18% respectively.

In 1989, 60% of children in custody belonged to racial or ethnic minority groups (approximately 42% African-American, 15% Hispanic, and 2% American Indian, Alaskan native, Asian, or Pacific Islander). The number of white juveniles held in public facilities decreased by 5% between 1987 and 1989, while the number of African-American and Hispanic juveniles increased by 14% and 10% respectively.

---

[i] OJJDP. January 1991. op cit.

Juveniles in Long-Term Facilities Report Extensive Alcohol and Other Drug Use, Less Likely to Receive School-Based HIV Prevention Due to Low High School Graduation Rates

In 1988, the Bureau of Justice Statistics, released a special report, Survey of Youth in Custody, 1987 which supplements the information provided by the biennial Children in Custody census. This report describes various characteristics of over 2,600 juveniles and young adults held in long-term, state-operated institutions. Youth in these facilities are generally more serious offenders with longer criminal records.[125]

The data included in this report (summaries of the youths' criminal histories, family structure, educational background, drug and alcohol use, and peer group activities) are particularly helpful for designing HIV and other prevention and health-related services for juvenile offenders.

In June 1992, OJJDP plans to consider a proposal to update and expand the contents of the Youth in Custody report.[126] Absent more recent data, Table 7 summarizes the extent of illegal drug use among youth in long-term state-operated juvenile facilities, one of the most dramatic findings of the Youth in Custody, 1987 report.

Table 7: Illegal Drug Use by Youth in Long-Term State-Operated Juvenile Institutions, Year End 1987[j]

Type of Drug	Ever Used Drugs	Used Regularly
Any drug	82.7%	63.1%
Marijuana/Hashish	81.2%	56.0%
Cocaine	46.1%	21.5%
Amphetamines	36.3%	15.5%
LSD	28.9%	11.9%
Barbiturates	27.3%	8.9%
PCP	22.6%	8.9%
Quaaludes	14.6%	3.0%
Heroin	13.0%	5.2%

Compared with surveys of high school students, drug use is not only more prevalent among incarcerated youth, but also begins at an earlier age. Among juvenile offenders who reported a history of drug use, the median age at onset was 12 years, with nearly one in five reporting drug use before age ten and 82% reporting major drug use (including heroin, cocaine, LSD, and PCP) before age 16.[127]

Three in four juvenile offenders surveyed reported drinking alcohol one or more times per week in the year before admission, and nearly half (48%) reported being under the influence of either alcohol or other drugs at the time of their current offense.

Survey of Youth in Custody, 1987 also found that juveniles in these institutions had significantly lower levels of education than comparable youth in the general population. In the general population, 76% of youth ages 15-17 had completed more than eight years of school, compared with only 42% of long-term juvenile facility residents. Less than 3% of youth in long-term, state-operated juvenile facilities were high school graduates.[128] Failure to complete high school reduces exposure to school-based

---

(j) BJS. 1988. op cit. Used regularly = used once per week or more for at least a month.

AIDS education, and thus increases risk.

Smaller Studies Confirm High Rates of Sexual Activity and Drug Use, Limited HIV-Related Knowledge Among Detained and Incarcerated Youth

Although the findings are not easily generalized, several studies of institutionalized adolescents provide additional evidence that these youth are at increased risk of HIV infection. In cooperation with the CDC, the National Commission on Correctional Health Care (NCCHC) has implemented a limited Youth Risk Behavior Survey in randomly selected juvenile facilities in five states, including Massachusetts, New York, Tennessee, Texas, and Wisconsin.[129] Survey questions cover a variety of behaviors, including sexual activity, use of alcohol and other substances, violence, and suicide.

Damon Marquis, Director of Health Education of the NCCHC, presented the preliminary results of the study in testimony submitted to the Select Committee. His summary of the results to date showed that:

- more than 90% reported having been sexually active; more than one-fourth reported having been pregnant or impregnating a sexual partner; and nearly six in ten (56%) reported not using a condom the last time they willingly engaged in sexual intercourse;

- more than 91% of respondents reported having consumed alcohol at least once, with 35% reporting having at least one drink of alcohol 100 or more days in their life; and,

- eighty-one percent of youth reported trying marijuana and 32% reported trying cocaine in some form, and 9% reported injecting drugs.[130]

Additional NCCHC findings suggest that suicidal behavior is significant among incarcerated youth. Nearly one-third reported seriously considering suicide, and one in five actually attempted suicide at least once in the previous year.

While providing compelling descriptions of many of the risks that these youth face, Marquis notes that, since analyses are preliminary, findings should not be generalized to all youth in juvenile facilities nationwide.[131]

A 1991 study compared AIDS-related knowledge, attitudes, and behaviors among incarcerated youth with adolescents in public schools in San Francisco.[132] While both groups demonstrated high levels of general knowledge about the transmission of AIDS, incarcerated youth were less likely to have information regarding risk-reduction strategies. Among youth enrolled in school, 85% correctly identified condom use as a means of reducing the risk of HIV transmission, compared with three-fourths of incarcerated youth. Moreover, only 62% of incarcerated youth (compared with 80% of school youth) recognized that sexual abstinence reduces the risk of HIV infection. Similarly, only 56% of incarcerated youth identified not having sexual partners who use intravenous drugs as a strategy to reduce risk of HIV transmission, compared with 72% of school youth. Incarcerated youth were significantly more likely to perceive themselves as susceptible to infection (69% vs. 45%).

Table 8 summarizes the substantial differences in sexual and drug-related behaviors between the two study groups. Youth in detention had engaged in the highest risk behaviors at more than three times the rate of youth enrolled in public school.

Table 8: Prevalence of Sexual and Drug-Related Behaviors Among Detained Youth and Youth Enrolled in Public School[k]

Behavior	Detention (n=113)	Enrolled in Public School (n=802)
Proportion Sexually Active	99.1%	28.3%
Number of Sexual Partners		
At Least Three (Lifetime)	84.4%	15.1%
At Least Two (Past Year)	72.9%	8.1%
Percent Reporting Age at First Sexual Intercourse Before or At 12 Years of Age	52.1%	25.9%
Proportion Reporting:		
Consistent Condom Use[l]	28.6%	37.3%
Use of Intravenous Drugs[m]	12.9%	3.7%

These findings are similar to those from a 1988 study which compared knowledge and attitudes about AIDS among nearly 1,600 urban, suburban, gay, and incarcerated youth. This study found that incarcerated youth demonstrated significantly poorer knowledge about AIDS, lower agreement with health guidelines, lower perceived personal threat, lower perceived norms about safer sex practices, and lower personal efficacy in avoiding infection than the other three groups studied.[133]

Several studies indicate that youth in correctional facilities initiate sexual activity earlier than their counterparts in the general population, and are more likely to have STDs. Hein, et al., found that the average age of first intercourse among females in one detention center (n=378) was 12 years.[134] Virtually all

(k) DiClemente, R.J., et al. "Comparison of AIDS Knowledge, Attitudes, and Behaviors Among Incarcerated Adolescents and a Public School Sample in San Francisco." American Journal of Public Health. Vol. 81. No. 5. May 1991. Table 3.

(l) Among sexually active, defined as always using condoms.

(m) Proportion reporting intravenous drug use at lease once.

females in this sample were sexually active. Rates of STDs in female juveniles ranged from 6% to 20% in various facilities.[135]

In one study of 306 incarcerated male youth, the median age of first intercourse was 11 years. Ninety-six percent were sexually active at the time of the study, 19% reported male/female anal sex, 14% had sex with an IV drug user, 11% had a history of STDs, and 37% reported never using condoms.[136]

A 1987 study of sexual activity and STDs by the Los Angeles County Department of Health Services, which had an average daily population of 1,850 minors, reported that 75% of the male population was sexually active, with high numbers of sexual partners. Three percent of males tested were found to have gonorrhea, and 13% had asymptomatic chlamydia. Among females, who represented 12% of the juvenile population, 98% were sexually active, 10% were pregnant at the time of the examination, 33% had chlamydia, 10% had gonorrhea, and 28% had trichomoniasis.[137]

High rates of STDs among female offenders illustrate a point made by a key informant in a Select Committee survey about the special needs of females which are often overlooked within the juvenile justice system:

> [We] make a special effort to reach out to girls who have often neglected themselves and have a difficult time dealing with partners...there is far less resistance on the part of males to at least say that using a condom is OK...girls are afraid to even bring the subject up...there is an exceptionally high probability that they will be infected by their older partners. Sex and babies are powerful ways to feel important to someone at least for a short time. The girls get STDs all the time and don't get treatment.[138]

Despite Clear Evidence of High-Risk Behavior, Medical and AIDS-Related Services for Juvenile Offenders Are Few and Largely Unevaluated

In 1990, the Council on Scientific Affairs of the American Medical Association found that youth who come to correctional facilities are a medically underserved population that often arrives with substantial existing physical and emotional problems caused by a variety of factors, including past physical or psychosocial insults, lifestyle habits, and lack of prior health care.[139]

As was noted previously, little is known about the quality and availability of primary and preventive health care to youth in custody. Studies indicate, however, that adult inmates are more likely than juvenile offenders to receive HIV education.[140] A 1988 study found that all adult prison inmates and approximately two-thirds of surveyed jail inmates received some AIDS education.[141] In the same year, the American Correctional Association (ACA) found that 14 state systems of juvenile correction provided no AIDS education for youth, and seven provided only staff training. Of the 29 detention facilities that responded to the ACA survey, nine provided no instruction for young offenders, and two provided no programming for staff.[142]

Moreover, the Select Committee is unaware of any systematic attempts to evaluate existing HIV prevention and related services programs in correctional facilities serving youth. This apparent failure is underscored by the lack of baseline data about high-risk behavior that is required to inform prevention planners. The Director of the National Institute of Justice, James Stewart, clarified specific information needs:

> Correctional administrators thus continue to face tough decisions about institutional management, the best and most equitable means of identifying and treating inmates with HIV disease, potential legal issues, and the costs of medical care. Policy makers and corrections officials cannot afford to wait until medical science produces an ultimate answer. To address the problem effectively today, they need the most accurate and up-to-date information available.[143]

Approaches that have been shown to be effective in public schools may not be useful with juvenile offenders. According to Gary Shostak, Director of Health Services for the Massachusetts Department of Youth services:

> It's difficult to measure the long-term impact of the [prevention] program...to know if what matters most is what is said, or who said it. It's difficult for adults who have little

in common with the youth to translate what they know into something the youth take to heart and make sense of for themselves.

One program that appears to have made progress overcoming this "culture gap" between juvenile offenders and adult AIDS educators was developed by YouthCare, Inc. for the Seattle-King County Department of Public Health. An evaluation of this program found that YouthCare's curriculum, which includes activities jointly designed by staff and detained youth, produced knowledge gains and increased intentions to behave safely.[144] Additional suggestions for effective ways to involve detained youth in program design have been offered,[145] but not evaluated.

In the absence of sufficient data about what works in reducing risk in juvenile offenders, an effort has been made to develop a general policy for serving these youth based on a consensus of experienced providers. The National Commission on Correctional Health Care has published standards to assist correctional facilities in designing HIV-related procedures. These standards include recommendations in the following policy areas: education and counseling; prevention; HIV-antibody testing and counseling; confidentiality; nondiscrimination/segregation in housing; and practice of universal precautions.[146]

Barriers to provision of AIDS services to juvenile offenders have also been identified by the NCCHC. These range from fear of contagion to inadequate agency policy. Suggestions for overcoming these barriers are NCCHC's Health Education Curriculum for Incarcerated Youth: Training Manual, and include, for example, networking with agencies experienced with HIV/AIDS issues and becoming educated about current health matters.[147]

Incarceration and Detention Present Unique Opportunities for Providing Prevention and Services to Hard-to-Reach Youth

Despite the challenges enumerated above, the period of incarceration or detention offers an important opportunity to provide medical assistance, including HIV prevention services, to troubled youth. In testimony submitted to the Select Committee, Marquis observed:

> Many of these youth have not received the benefit of conventional health educational resources because they were out of school and/or homeless and/or runaways prior to being placed in juvenile facilities. For others, this may be the only time a proactive health education program is offered in any setting. This is an excellent opportunity to provide the youth with the information and resources necessary to make vital behavior changes.[148]

Thus, child welfare and epidemiological considerations converge to emphasize the critical importance of addressing the HIV prevention and other health care needs of detained and incarcerated youth.

D. HIV-RELATED NEEDS OF YOUTH IN FOSTER CARE

There are no reliable estimates of the prevalence of HIV among adolescents in foster care. Because states vary considerably in their collection and reporting of data on children in foster care, and no central, Federal data collection system exists, little is known about the adolescents who are placed in out-of-home care. In its 1990 report No Place to Call Home: Discarded Children in America, the Select Committee found that foster care data collection requires significant improvement.[149]

Various studies indicate that youth in foster care are at increased risk of unprotected sexual activity and alcohol and other drug use; however, these youth rarely have access to HIV prevention curricula or related services. Barriers to providing HIV prevention and services to youth in foster care include lack of placements, funding and liability issues, and confusion about who should provide HIV-related services.

The Extent of HIV Among Youth in Foster Care May Be Underestimated

The most recent estimate of the number of HIV-infected children in foster care is based on 1989 data collected by DHHS.

DHHS found that more than 800 children with HIV had been placed in foster care homes. However, the number of adolescents within this population was not estimated.[150] Child welfare and related agencies do not conduct routine HIV testing and have minimal knowledge of the HIV infection status of adolescents in their care. Only infants and children exposed to HIV through maternal infection, sexual abuse by an infected adult, or blood transfusion, or adolescents with a known risk factor such as injected drug use, are typically tested.[151]

Adolescents in Foster Care Engage in Risky Behavior That May Lead to HIV Infection

While data are incomplete, it appears that many youth in foster care react to the stress and discontinuity of out-of-home placement by exhibiting behavior that can increase exposure to HIV. A survey conducted in the Midwest indicates that child-welfare clients have high rates of premarital sexual activity and low rates of contraceptive use, suggesting a high risk of HIV infection.[152] Among females ages 13-18, child welfare clients were 50% more likely to report having had sex than females from a national sample. This study also found that females in the foster care system reported a history of pregnancy twice as often, were less knowledgeable about birth control and sexuality than similar females who were living at home, and that 48% had experienced some form of sexual abuse.[153] (See "Considerations for Serving Youth Who Have Been Sexually Abused" in this chapter for further analysis of these issues.)

Many youth enter the foster care system because they have run away. Once placed, these youth may be more likely to run away than young people who live with their natural parents.[154] (See "HIV-Related Needs of Runaway and Homeless Youth" in this chapter for further analysis of these issues.)

Most adolescents leave the foster care system via "emancipation," i.e., they reach an age beyond which the state no longer offers services. Little is known about where these adolescents go upon leaving the foster care system,[155] or about their continued risk of HIV infection, but preliminary findings are alarming.

Under contract with DHHS, Westat, Inc. studied the needs of youth emancipated from the foster care system and found that 17 percent had drug abuse problems and nine percent had some other unspecified health problem. Seventeen percent of the females were pregnant.[156]

Barriers to HIV Prevention for Youth in the Foster Care System

Few Foster Placements Available for Teens

Of the 340,000 individuals thought to be in foster care on a given day in 1988, 36.5% were over the age of 13.[157] Preliminary projections indicate that the foster care population exceeded 400,000 in 1990.[158] Despite the fact that more than 100,000 teens needed foster care placement in 1988, the numbers of available placements for this group have continued to decline.[159] According to the Child Welfare League of America (CWLA), "workers report greatest difficulty finding placements for teenagers because foster parents are uncomfortable with having sexually active teens in their homes."[160] In addition, the foster care system allocates most of its severely limited resources towards protection and placement of infants and young children; compared with adolescents, young children are seen as less able to escape abuse or to care for themselves.[161]

It is especially difficult to find foster families willing and able to cope with the health care needs of adolescents who are infected with HIV. In the case of one young man diagnosed with AIDS, a local social service agency contacted over 200 different organizations before finding a placement.[162] Subsequently, the same agency (Professional Parenting of North Carolina) found placements for two infants with AIDS and concluded:

> We would offer that the difficulty an agency faces in placing teens with AIDS is far greater than that of placing and managing infected toddlers...it is that teens...evoke realistic fears concerning sex and drugs, and, because of their relative

mobility, they also inherently present far greater monitoring and management complexities.[163]

Adults seeking to become foster parents of children with HIV infection are screened carefully and undergo special counseling and education. Service agencies and advocacy organizations have developed recruitment tools to educate potential foster parents about HIV disease and about the care of children who have HIV-infection or AIDS. To date, however, federally funded efforts have targeted infant placement.[164]

Funding and Liability Issues Starting to Emerge

Families willing to provide foster care for HIV-infected youth face serious problems with reimbursement. Foster care payments are insufficient and delayed, even for children without special medical needs,[165] and the situation is further complicated for teenagers who, as a group, have inadequate access to appropriate medical services.[166]

The Medicaid program is the primary means for paying the costs of health care for children with HIV disease or AIDS who are in the child welfare system. However, states have considerable discretion regarding the content and coverage of their Medicaid plans. Certain drugs and procedures, for example, may or may not be covered by states.[167] (See Chapter IV.)

Child welfare experts report that progress in the development of policy specifically relevant to AIDS has been made in some states. By 1988, at least 21 states had begun to develop adoption and foster care policies for children with AIDS.[168] By July 1989, 18 states had established higher reimbursement rates for foster children who are HIV infected or who have AIDS (AR, CA, CT, DE, FL, GA, ID, KY, ME, MD, NE, NJ, NM, NY, RI, SC, TN, WV).[169]

According to CWLA state foster care agencies most frequently request assistance and training related to policy recommendations and standards for HIV-infected individuals.[170] Existing state policies often only address issues of sex education rather than HIV prevention, while HIV-specific policies most often address issues related to infection control, confidentiality, HIV testing, rules for foster care placement, adoption, group care, and staff and foster parent training. Arizona, however, has developed a more extensive policy that includes the provision of "age appropriate" client education services that address both sexuality and infection control procedures.[171]

The most pressing liability issues for child welfare departments involve testing for antibodies to HIV and disclosure of HIV status.[172] State policies for children and youth in state care are typically patterned after those designed to protect adults from discrimination.[173] Some child welfare advocates argue however, that more flexible standards would be appropriate for children and youth.[174] Because the issues around "need to know" depend to some extent on the age of the child, it may not be advisable to have uniform policies that address children and youth.[175]

Confidentiality issues involve both foster care and other "third party" adults, including school officials and other service providers. For example, many child welfare advocates fear that the secrecy surrounding the HIV status of children may adversely affect decision-making about health care and impede recruitment efforts for foster care and adoptive parents.[176] In cases when HIV-infected children are asymptomatic, the foster parents' need to know depends on their responsibilities for the health and protection of children in their care. For example, the foster parent may not need to know the HIV status of the child or adolescent if the placement is short term and the youth does not require medical or other services during that time.[177]

While questions remain, most public agency adoption and foster care specialists believe that state regulations and policies implemented to date afford sufficient flexibility to allow for communication of necessary information to those with a legitimate need to know.[178]

Confusion About Responsibility for AIDS-Related Education Remains Widespread

Despite the evidence that children in foster care may be at

very high risk of unintended pregnancy and sexually transmitted diseases, states fail to maintain the records necessary to plan for family planning and educational services. For example, in 1987, no state knew the number of adolescents in foster care who had become pregnant while in the state's custody.[179]

Since adolescents in foster care frequently move from placement to placement, they often find themselves in new communities where they have no close ties with service providers or other caregivers. Teens in new foster homes may not feel comfortable enough to seek advice actively, especially advice about sexuality and other behaviors associated with HIV risk.[180]

There is little agreement about who has the right, responsibility, or obligation to talk to teens in foster care about sex, drugs and AIDS. Is it the responsibility of foster parents, caseworkers, the school system, or the biological parents?[181]

One study conducted in Wisconsin found that 48% of foster homes, 32% of group homes, and 21% of other child-caring institutions were unclear about their legal right to provide birth control information without parental consent.[182] Two-thirds of caseworkers surveyed in this study believed that providing birth control information to teens in their care was the responsibility of foster parents rather than their own. At the same time, few foster parents (less than 25%) spoke to their sexually active teens directly about sexual issues or referred them to a physician or family planning provider. Others argue that the responsibility for providing sexuality education and advice about family planning to adolescents in foster care continues to rest with the biological parents, even when the child has been removed from that home.[183]

Because of the ambiguity of relevant policy, and because adults tend to be uncomfortable talking to teens about sexuality, HIV/AIDS education for children in foster care is haphazard at best. Anecdotal information collected from child welfare administrators in the early 1980s indicated that few agency leaders had given adequate consideration to their responsibility to ensure the provision of sexual guidance to youth in their care.[184] In 1986, researchers surveyed foster care administrators in 48 states about their sex education and family planning services and found that virtually no state had dealt with these issues in a comprehensive manner. Only nine states had any formal written policy concerning sex education for foster care clients. Twenty-nine states offered special training in teen sexuality to foster care parents, but only five mandated that parents actually receive it. Nineteen states offered this training to their caseworkers, but it was mandated in only four states.[185]

In the overburdened foster care system, controversial topics are often ignored until a problem arises. For example, discussions about a foster child's sexuality are often avoided until after she or he has become sexually active.[186] Similarly, according to CWLA, the foster care system neglects HIV prevention. Although CWLA guidelines recommend training for all foster parents, group home staff, and adolescents in care, HIV education is too often provided only when clients or family members are infected.[187]

Needs of Gay and Lesbian Youth and the Role of Males in Prevention Efforts Often Ignored in Foster Care System

There is no accurate information about how many gay and lesbian youth are in foster care, but special challenges attendant to provision of services to this group have been noted. "Gay and lesbian youth are often not placeable. The few who find placement are often sent back. We want to provide a safe place for them, where their sexuality won't be an issue."[188] Despite the shortage of placement settings, exacerbated in the instance of HIV-infected gay youth, many agencies do not allow homosexual adults to become foster parents.[189]

In addition, the few prevention efforts currently underway in the foster care system are aimed almost exclusively at young women.[190] As noted by J. Burt Annin of CWLA, the sexuality education needs of males are largely ignored, perhaps as a function of a widespread lack of male leadership in child welfare, or of the perception that females bear the responsibility of sexual activity in the case of pregnancy, or of homophobia.[191] Whatever the cause, such a service shortfall ignores the risk of contracting HIV and other sexually transmitted diseases faced by males in foster care.

Guidelines for HIV/AIDS Education for Foster Care Clients Exist

Some counties have developed programs to address teen sexuality and HIV-related issues of foster care clients. For example, Family and Children's Services of Chattanooga, Tennessee, received a grant from the Hamilton County Health Department to provide sexuality education services for "unadoptable teens" living in group homes. Several three-day courses were held on topics including: teen pregnancy, negotiation skills, human anatomy, STDs, and HIV/AIDS.[192]

The Institute for the Study of Children and Families at Eastern Michigan University, under a grant from the DHHS has published national guidelines for HIV/AIDS and sexuality education of adolescents in foster care. The guidelines are a module of a larger independent living skills curriculum entitled Choices and Consequences. They include a hands-on workbook designed to be completed by the adolescents and their parents or caregivers, and deal with topics ranging from choosing to postpone sexual relations to homosexuality. By July 1991, Choices and Consequences had been disseminated to agencies in 32 states.[193]

Another model curriculum, the Safe Choices Guide produced by the National Network of Runaway and Youth Services, includes a unit to train foster parents about educating young people in their care regarding AIDS and HIV prevention.[194] The unit describes foster parents' responsibilities to provide this kind of information, addresses how parents can be effective AIDS educators, and discusses the needs of foster families who care for HIV-infected youth.

Additional information for families and other caregivers is available in Initial Guidelines and Meeting the Challenge of HIV Infection in Family Foster Care published by the Child Welfare League of America.[195]

Role of the Federal Government Limited to Basic Child Welfare Services, Ignores Needs of Teens for HIV Prevention and Services

Child welfare services are provided through state, local and private agencies, with Federal Government support accounting for an estimated 40% of the total costs of the child welfare system.[196] Federal support for child welfare services is primarily authorized by Title IV-B (child welfare services) and Title IV-E (foster care and adoption assistance) of the Social Security Act. Because of minimal reporting requirements, there are no specific data on the services provided by the states under Title IV-B. Title IV-E provides maintenance payments to be used for food, shelter, clothing, daily supervision, school supplies, personal incidentals, liability insurance for the child, and reasonable travel to the child's home for visits. In addition, the Social Services Block Grant under Title XX of the Social Security Act provides some financial assistance although specific activities are not reported.[197]

The Abandoned Infants Assistance Act is another Federal effort established to respond to the problems associated with substance-abusing parents, and the increase in the number of boarder babies in hospitals, particularly, those with AIDS. Although the program recruits and trains foster families for these infants and young children, it is not required by law to include services for adolescents.

While beyond the scope of this report, reforms needed in the foster care system as a whole have been detailed in a 1990 publication of the Select Committee entitled: No Place to Call Home: Discarded Children in America. Specific Federal policy recommendations have been offered by the Child Welfare League of America, and are appended to the League's aforementioned guidelines.

E. HIV-RELATED NEEDS OF YOUTH ALREADY USING ALCOHOL AND OTHER DRUGS

HIV-related drug behavior in youth encompasses more than intravenous (IV) drug use. While IV drug use can transmit HIV directly, the use of other drugs may increase the likelihood of unsafe sexual behaviors by lowering inhibitions, and adversely altering judgment.[198] Moreover, some drug-using adolescents exchange sex for drugs. Frequently, their partners are drug users and drug dealers who have had multiple sex partners and who are at high risk of having been exposed to HIV.[199]

Model demonstration drug prevention programs illustrate that in order to have a positive impact on adolescent drug use, an education program needs to be incorporated into a comprehensive program that encompasses peer pressure resistance, parental and community involvement, and media participation.

Little effort has been expended to include the increased risk of HIV exposure with drug use in school-based prevention curricula. Instead, HIV/AIDS education, when provided, is usually taught separately. Moreover, many HIV prevention classes focus only on the dissemination of information, and few mention the fact that use of alcohol and other drugs can increase a teen's risk for HIV exposure.

For teens who are drug users, barriers to treatment (including a critical shortage of treatment programs and too few school-based early intervention programs) impede efforts to reduce high-risk behaviors for both drug use and HIV. Moreover, little is known about the effectiveness of drug treatment in the elimination of drug use.

Behaviors That Place Drug-Using Teens at Risk of HIV

Injecting Drug Use

In roughly one in eight diagnosed AIDS cases among teens, injecting drug use (IDU)[(n)] has been implicated as a risk

---

[(n)] Because HIV can be transmitted by injecting drugs under the skin or into muscle, i.e. with heroin use and steroid use, CDC recently changed its terminology for AIDS case reporting from "intravenous drug user" to "injecting drug user." In this report, when citing data reported as intravenous drug use, the original terminology is maintained. (CDC. HIV/AIDS Prevention Newsletter. Vol.2. No.2. October 1991.)

factor.[200] Among females ages 13-19 who have been diagnosed with AIDS, 28% of the cases are related to injecting drug use.[201] The widely prevalent ritual of sharing apparatus to inject illicit drugs appears to be the central vector of transmission; a National Academy of Sciences report found that sharing needles and "works" is most common at the earliest stages of IV drug use.[202] Although most drug use among teens does not involve injection, 10% of those in drug abuse treatment programs who reported IV drug use during the previous year were age 21 or younger.[203]

While drug use declined overall from 1985-1991, data from the National Household Survey conducted by the National Institute on Drug Abuse (NIDA) show that in 1991, approximately 1% of youth ages 12-17 and 2.3% of young adults ages 18-25 have injected illicit drugs.[204] In a large national secondary school survey, two percent of students ages 13-18 reported having ever shared needles.[205] In both the National Household Survey and the secondary school survey, males were twice as likely as females to engage in this HIV-related drug behavior. Racial and ethnic differences in adolescent drug injection behavior are not substantial. Youth who do not complete high school and those who live in metropolitan areas use IV drugs at significantly higher rates than others in their age groups.[206]

Even higher estimates of injectable drug use come from the most recent NIDA High School Senior Survey.[207] Of the respondents in this large study, 2.9% reported the use of steroids (which are injected by 99% of users), and 1.3% reported heroin use. Additional injection-based risk is suggested by the non-crack cocaine use reported in the Senior Survey (9.4%). This figure closely parallels the estimate generated by the CDC's Youth Risk Behavior Survey estimate (9.3% of seniors).[208] However, neither of these sources analyzed the proportion of reported cocaine use that actually involved injection, and cocaine can be ingested in other ways.

Crack Cocaine Use

More than three in one hundred high school seniors report having used crack, and use of this drug is likely to be more prevalent among out-of-school youth. Crack use is believed to play an important role in fueling the HIV epidemic.[209] As described in Chapter I, one study of 13-19 year old African-American crack users in San Francisco and Oakland found that 96% were sexually active, 51% engaged in sexual activity while high on crack, and 25% of both males and females exchanged sexual favors for drugs or money.[210] The risk of unsafe sexual practices under such conditions is considerable; it is highly unlikely that the HIV serostatus, sex history, or drug habits of a partner would be known, and rare that condoms would be used. In this study, only 26% of males and 18% of females reported the use of condoms during their most recent sexual encounter.[211]

Alcohol Consumption

According to NIDA's 1990 High School Senior Survey, more than 90% of all American high school seniors have tried alcohol.[212] The majority of students took their first drink before they were 13 years old. A 1991 national survey of junior and senior high school students conducted by the Office of the Inspector General found that the average student who drinks is 16 years old and in the 10th grade.[213] More importantly, one in every three students reported drinking weekly, and one in four students had experienced a "binge" of five or more drinks in a row in the month prior to the survey. It is clear from these data that many adolescents not only drink, but do so frequently and excessively.

Alcohol facilitates unsafe sexual behaviors.[214] In a Massachusetts survey of youth ages 16-19, sexually active teens who drank were significantly less likely to use condoms.[215] Moreover, 16% of teens who had sex after drinking used condoms less often after drinking than when they had sex without drinking alcohol.

Barriers to Treatment for Drug Using Teens Remain

The initial identification of an adolescent with a drug-use problem is usually made by family and friends. Because most adolescents spend a large part of their day in school, teachers and peers may be the first to recognize an emerging problem.

Thus, school-based programs for the identification and referral of adolescent drug users and those at high risk for drug abuse seem to hold promise.[216] Student assistance programs, which are modeled on employee assistance programs, provide an example of school-based early intervention services including identification of students with problems, referral to other services in the community and, in some cases, the use of peer or guidance counselors already involved with other school programs.[217] In many communities, student assistance programs are one of the few drug abuse intervention programs available to economically disadvantaged students.[218] Many school systems view substance abuse as a health problem which is not germane to education, and often are reluctant to become involved.[219] In addition, students with drug problems may be unwilling to seek school-based services if they fear suspension for drug use.[220]

Another barrier to providing drug treatment for adolescents is the lack of valid assessment tools to identify which adolescents need treatment, and, if treatment is needed, what is appropriate. NIDA recently developed a comprehensive assessment and referral manual for adolescents which is undergoing further testing.[221]

Severe Shortages of Drug, Alcohol, and Methadone Treatment Programs for Teens Impede Successful HIV Prevention

There is a dire shortage of drug abuse treatment services for teens. The National Association of State Alcohol and Drug Abuse Directors have identified adolescents as the age group most in need of additional service slots.[222] Survey data from 1989 showed that at least 1,600,000 adolescents in the U.S. needed treatment for alcohol and drug abuse; however only 123,500 received it that year.[223]

Because there are few drug treatment programs specifically for adolescents, youth seldom receive drug abuse treatment in age-appropriate settings. Typically, teens are placed in treatment programs designed for adults or intended for younger children. Only 15% of adolescents being treated for alcohol use problems are in an adolescent-tailored treatment program, while nearly 25% are in treatment programs in which more than 90% of the treatment population is adults.[224]

Among adult IV drug users, methadone treatment programs have been an effective strategy in reducing the spread of HIV.[225] Methadone treatment involves the substitution of an orally administered synthetic narcotic for IV heroin. For this reason, admission to methadone treatment programs is usually limited to IV drug users who have failed other treatment modalities.[226] Although the use of methadone by adolescent IV drug users may be problematic because of legal and financial barriers, public health concerns could be well served by targeting this group. New IV drug users are the most likely group to share needles, and HIV seroprevalence is lowest among IV drug users who have been using injectable drugs for less than five years.[227]

The Effectiveness of Adolescent Treatment Programs Remains Uncertain

As noted above, drug and alcohol use plays a major role in the transmission of HIV infection among adolescents. For this reason, the availability of age-appropriate, effective drug treatment programs is a cornerstone in the prevention of adolescent HIV infection. Controversy exists regarding when and if an adolescent requires treatment for drug abuse, the efficacy and effectiveness of various kinds of treatment, the length of treatment and the type of treatment setting.[228] In 1990, a National Academy of Science committee study on drug treatment concluded that little was known about drug treatment effectiveness for adolescents, and recommended that drug treatment of adolescents be studied intensively.[229]

Available drug abuse treatment services include self-help groups, outpatient treatment, residential treatment and inpatient treatment. Self-help groups and outpatient treatment are usually targeted at teens who are highly motivated and who have either successfully completed an inpatient or residential treatment program, or have not received prior treatment. Strategies may include education, counseling, social skills development, psychotherapy, family therapy and self-help. Residential and inpatient treatment programs typically serve teens who are less motivated and have not responded to outpatient therapy. In addition to the strategies offered in outpatient treatment, these programs offer a therapeutic environment and daily supervision.[230]

The effectiveness of drug treatment requires further study. Specifically, definitive research is needed to determine when outpatient or inpatient treatment is most effective.[231] Two large studies in which inpatient and outpatient treatments were compared resulted in contradictory results.[232] A study of delinquent and drug abusing teens randomly assigned to inpatient or outpatient treatment noted similar improvement in behavior in both groups.[233] In most studies, short-term gains are reported, but sustained abstinence has not been clearly demonstrated.[234]

Existing Programs for Drug and HIV Prevention Still Few, But Expanding

Largest Federal Effort, Drug Free Schools, Fails to Mention Drug Link to HIV Risk

The largest federally funded drug prevention program for youth is the Drug Free Schools program mandated in every state (P.L.99-570). As a condition of eligibility for Federal funds, local educational agencies must certify that they have adopted and implemented a firm drug policy (P.L.101-226). The Drug Free Schools and Communities Act Amendments of 1989 state that, at a minimum, a prevention program must convey to the students that the use of illicit drugs and the unlawful possession and use of alcohol is wrong and harmful; include standards of conduct that clearly prohibit the unlawful possession, use, or distribution of illicit drugs and alcohol by students on school premises or as a part of any school activities; and include a clear statement that sanctions will be imposed on students who violate the standards of conduct.[235]

The Department of Education's interpretation of the statute is that schools should adopt a "no-use" policy.[236] As a result, the Department of Education has refused requests to include information regarding HIV-related risk behaviors in their drug prevention curriculum, despite leeway in the statute and the encouragement of the Office of Substance Abuse Prevention to do so.[237] By emphasizing a "no use" policy, schools may alienate many students already involved with drugs, particularly alcohol. Goodstadt noted that a "no use" approach ignores the realities of use.[238] For adolescents already using alcohol and other drugs, setting intermediate goals that reduce use as a first step toward ultimately eliminating drug use may be more appropriate.[239]

To date, there are no data to show that the Drug-Free School Programs are effective in reducing the frequency with which adolescents use drugs.[240]

State and Local Resources for Comprehensive Approaches Limited

By June 1991, 31 states and the District of Columbia had mandated AIDS education in the public schools.[241] Because local communities determine the content and scope of the school curriculum, there is no standard format for the delivery of HIV education and associated high-risk behaviors. In fact, a review of 18 AIDS curricula by CDC staff showed that the majority of programs were only one-hour or one-class in duration, and few (four of 18) emphasized that specific behaviors, including injecting drugs, place an individual at risk for AIDS.[242] To be most effective in deterring or changing high-risk behaviors, education about HIV and associated high-risk behaviors needs to be taught within a comprehensive health or family life curriculum.[243] Currently, only 19 states require that HIV education be taught in this manner.[244]

Preliminary Results of Programs for Out-of-School Youth Promising

Agencies have begun developing programs to provide comprehensive and appropriate information on HIV to teens who have dropped out of school.[245] In addition, NIDA sponsors a number of demonstration projects designed to provide HIV education and risk reduction interventions to injecting drug users, including adolescents, who are not in drug treatment programs. Preliminary data on adult IV drug users served by these demonstration projects show a reduction in unsafe sexual and drug use practices.[246] Data on adolescents have yet to be analyzed.

Few Model Alcohol and Other Drug Prevention Programs Exist

No single intervention has proved effective in preventing drug abuse.[247] The most promising strategies are peer education/training programs and, for high-risk youth, programs that provide alternatives to drug use such as community activities, remedial tutoring, and individual skill building activities.[248] Researchers emphasize that an effective program requires a comprehensive community effort that targets many of the major social influences on youth, including school, parents, community organizations and the media.[249]

An example of a comprehensive drug prevention program is Project STAR (Students Taught Awareness and Resistance).[250] The program, which serves students in the Kansas City metropolitan area schools, supplements training in peer pressure resistance skills with parental involvement, parent-child communications training, involving community leaders in the organization of a drug abuse prevention task force, and mass media programming of drug prevention. The school-based educational component is taught to sixth and seventh grade students, and booster sessions are provided annually through grade 12. Results at one and two years among students from a wide variety of socioeconomic and drug risk groups show that the expected increase in alcohol and marijuana use was reduced by 20% and 30% respectively. The frequency of other drug use was not evaluated.

Project I-STAR (Indiana Students Taught Awareness and Resistance) in Indianapolis is modeled closely on Project STAR. Based on the early evaluations of Project STAR, the Indiana curriculum includes three additional lessons about alcohol as a drug. Preliminary evaluation data from I-STAR indicate that students who did not participate in the program were 21% more likely to increase their use of alcohol and 25% more likely to increase their use of marijuana than students who did participate in the program.[251]

F. HIV-RELATED NEEDS OF RACIAL AND ETHNIC MINORITY ADOLESCENTS

Like adults, racial and ethnic minority adolescents are at a disproportionately higher risk of AIDS than their white peers. What is known about risk behaviors, attitudes and beliefs of minority adolescents suggests that special preventive interventions targeting this group are urgently needed. Such interventions must be culturally competent, cognizant of special geographic and economic barriers to serving minority youth, and continually refined by feedback from the target population.[252] Evaluation of the effectiveness of promising preventive programs for minority adolescents is long overdue.

Seventy Percent of Female Adolescents with AIDS Are Minority, Modes of HIV Transmission Same for White and Racial and Ethnic Minority Youth

As detailed in Chapter I, the pattern of AIDS cases among youth is different from the adult pattern.[253] A key difference is the greater proportion of minority cases among those ages 13-24. While for adults (over age 25) the majority of reported AIDS cases (by the end of 1991) were among non-Hispanic whites (55%), the majority of AIDS cases reported in those ages 20-24 have been among racial and ethnic minority youth (55%). An even larger proportion (58%) of AIDS cases have been diagnosed among minority youth ages 13-19.

A closer examination of AIDS case data for youth ages 13-19 reveals that among females with AIDS, 71% are minority, as shown in Table 9.

Table 9: AIDS Cases Among Youth Ages 13-19 by Race/Ethnicity Through 1991[(o)]

Race/Ethnicity	Males #	(%)	Females #	(%)	Total #	(%)
White	271	(47%)	61	(29%)	332	(42%)
Other Races/Ethnicities:						
African American	175	(30%)	117	(55%)	292	(37%)
Hispanic	119	(21%)	32	(15%)	151	(19%)
Asian/Pac. Island	7	(1%)	1	(<1%)	8	(1%)
Native American/ AK Native	5	(1%)	1	(<1%)	6	(1%)
All	577	(100%)	212	(100%)	789	(100%)

As described previously, young adults and teens are more likely to have contracted AIDS through heterosexual transmission or contaminated blood than are those over age 25. They are less likely than adults to have been infected as a result of homosexual activity. Among youth ages 13-19, three cases of AIDS are reported in males for each case in females, a much lower ratio than in adults (roughly 9 men to 1 woman).[254]

Tables 10 and 11 describe the modes of HIV transmission among teens in greater detail than was presented in Chapter I of this report and highlight differences by gender and racial and ethnic groups.

(o) Special data request prepared by Reporting and Analysis Section, Surveillance Branch, Centers for Disease Control. January 13, 1992.

Table 10: AIDS Cases Among Males, Ages 13-19, By Race/Ethnicity and Mode of Transmission, Reported Through 1991[p]

Mode of Transmission	White #	White (%)	African-American #	African-American (%)	Hispanic #	Hispanic (%)	Asian/Pac. Islander #	Asian/Pac. Islander (%)	Amer. Indian/Alaskan Native #	Amer. Indian/Alaskan Native (%)
Men Having Sex with Men	63	(23%)	97	(55%)	35	(29%)	1	(14%)	1	(20%)
Injecting Drug Use	10	(4%)	12	(7%)	22	(18%)	0	(-0-)	0	(-0-)
Men Having Sex with Men and Injecting Drugs	10	(4%)	10	(6%)	12	(10%)	0	(-0-)	1	(20%)
Hemophilia/Coag. Disorder	165	(61%)	27	(15%)	38	(32%)	5	(71%)	3	(60%)
Heterosexual Contact	0	(-0-)	12	(7%)	0	(-0-)	0	(-0-)	0	(-0-)
Recpt. of Blood Transf., etc.	16	(6%)	5	(3%)	5	(4%)	1	(14%)	0	(-0-)
Other/Undetermined	7	(3%)	12	(7%)	7	(6%)	0	(-0-)	0	(-0-)
Total	**271**		**175**		**119**		**7**		**5**	

(p) Special Data request prepared by Reporting and Analysis Section, Surveillance Branch, Centers for Disease Control. January 13, 1992. Totals for percents may not add to 100 due to rounding. Note that of the 12 cases of AIDS among African-American males that were due to heterosexual transmission, 8 were due to being born in a Caribbean or sub-Sharan country or having sex with a female from one of these countries where most of the reported cases occur in heterosexuals and the male-to-female ratio is approximately 1:1.

Table 11: AIDS Cases Among Females, Ages 13-19, By Race/Ethnicity and Mode of Transmission, Reported Through 1991[q]

Mode of Transmission	White		African-American		Hispanic		Asian/Pac. Islander		Amer. Indian/Alaskan Native	
	#	(%)	#	(%)	#	(%)	#	(%)	#	(%)
Men Having Sex with Men	na	na	na	na	na	na	na	na	na	na
Injecting Drug Use	17	(28%)	29	(25%)	10	(31%)	1	(100%)	0	(-0-)
Men Having Sex with Men and Injecting Drugs	na	na	na	na	na	na	na	na	na	na
Hemophilia/Coag. Disorder	2	(3%)	1	(1%)	0	(-0-)	0	(-0-)	0	(-0-)
Heterosexual Contact	22	(36%)	61	(52%)	12	(38%)	0	(-0-)	1	(100%)
Recpt. of Blood Transf., etc.	14	(23%)	7	(6%)	5	(16%)	0	(-0-)	0	(-0-)
Other/Undetermined	6	(10%)	19	(16%)	4	(13%)	0	(-0-)	0	(-0-)
Total	61		117		32		1		1	

[q] Special Data request prepared by Reporting and Analysis Section, Surveillance Branch, Centers for Disease Control. January 13, 1992. Totals for percents may not add to 100 due to rounding.

Unlike racial differences in transmission patterns observed in adults, an examination of transmission routes as they vary by race and ethnic group among teens reveals only one marked difference -- white males are more likely to be infected as a result of hemophilia. If hemophilia is excluded from the list of transmission vectors, percentages of white and minority youth infected by drug use and same-gender sexual activity are very similar, especially among males. (See Table 12.)

Table 12: Noniatrogenic AIDS Cases Among Males, Ages 13-19, By Race/Ethnicity and Mode of Transmission, Reported Through 1991[r]

Mode of Transmission	White #	White (%)	African-American #	African-American (%)	Hispanic #	Hispanic (%)	Asian/Pac. Islander #	Asian/Pac. Islander (%)	Amer. Indian/ Alaskan Native #	Amer. Indian/ Alaskan Native (%)
Men Having Sex with Men	63	(70%)	97	(68%)	35	(46%)	1	(100%)	1	(50%)
Injecting Drug Use	10	(11%)	12	(8%)	22	(29%)	0	(-0-)	0	(-0-)
Men Having Sex with Men and Injecting Drugs	10	(11%)	10	(7%)	12	(16%)	0	(-0-)	1	(50%)
Heterosexual Contact	0	(-0-)	12	(8%)	0	(-0-)	0	(-0-)	0	(-0-)
Other/Undetermined	7	(8%)	12	(8%)	7	(9%)	0	(-0-)	0	(-0-)
Total	**90**		**143**		**76**		**1**		**2**	

(r) Special Data request prepared by Reporting and Analysis Section, Surveillance Branch, Centers for Disease Control. January 13, 1992. Totals for percents may not add to 100 due to rounding. Note that of the 12 cases of AIDS among African-American males that were due to heterosexual transmission, 8 were due to being born in a Caribbean or sub-Sharan country or having sex with a female from one of these countries where most of the reported cases occur in heterosexuals and the male-to-female ratio is approximately 1:1.

Information on Prevalence of HIV, High-Risk Sexual Behavior Shows Minority Youth to Be at Increased Risk

No national prevalence data exist regarding HIV infection in adolescents; however, data on military recruits and Job Corps applicants suggest that racial and ethnic minority youth, particularly African-American youth, are infected at significantly higher rates than white youth. (See Chapter I.) This increased risk parallels high rates of risky sexual behavior among African-American teens. As noted by the Office of Technology Assessment:

> There are significant differences between black and white adolescents in sexual activity, pregnancy, abortion, and childbearing rates. Black adolescents, many of whom are from socio-economically disadvantaged families, tend to initiate sexual activity at an earlier age, are less likely to use contraceptives, are more likely to experience out-of-wedlock births, and are less likely to have an abortion. Researchers disagree on the relative importance of socioeconomic status and other factors in accounting for these racial differences.[255]

According to one expert, all minority adolescent groups (African-American, Latino, Asian/Pacific Islander, and Native American) have higher rates of adolescent AIDS than whites.[256] In addition, white teens have a lower incidence of gonorrhea, syphilis, and genital herpes than African-American adolescents, the result of the same unprotected sexual activity that transmits HIV infection.[257]

Similarly, while the percentage of African-American and Hispanic youth that have ever used illicit drugs is smaller than that of white youth, indicators of heavy use show that both males and females from these minority groups are at increased risk. Compared with white youth, more African-American and Hispanic adolescents and young adults have used cocaine, crack and needles in the last month.[258] (See "HIV-Related Needs of Youth Already Using Alcohol or Other Drugs" in this chapter for further analysis of these issues.)

As noted above, studies of condom use in African-American teens have repeatedly shown that their usage is lower than that of white adolescents. However, when one recent study of 403 San Francisco teens controlled for the number of sexual partners and the perceived costs and benefits of condoms, no racial/ethnic differences in condom use were observed.[259]

Less is known about sexual and drug-related behaviors in youth from other racial and ethnic minority populations. However, one recent study of over 14,000 rural Native American students in grades 7-12 found that 35% of males and 27% of females reported having had sexual intercourse.[260] By grade 12, 65% of males and 57% of females reported being sexually experienced. Rates of contraceptive use were low among those students who were sexually active. Among students in grades 7-9, 36% of males and 57% of females reported using no method of contraception. By grades 10-12, 25% of sexually active males and 39% of sexually active females still reported no contraception. Among sexually experienced youth who did use contraceptives, 49% of males and 24% of females reported using only condoms.[261]

Minority Teens Know How HIV Is Transmitted But Have Misconceptions About How to Protect Themselves

Culturally "universal" solutions ignore emerging evidence that HIV prevention efforts have not been as effective with minority youth as with whites. Ethnic and racial differences in knowledge, attitudes, beliefs and behaviors relevant to risk of HIV infection have been documented, both between and within racial and ethnic groups. As outlined below, researchers have come to different conclusions about whether levels of general AIDS knowledge vary by race and ethnicity, but several experts have shown that certain dangerous misconceptions, attitudes and behaviors are more typical of minority youth.

A study conducted in San Francisco in 1985 found that white adolescents were more knowledgeable than African-American youth about the cause, transmission, and prevention of AIDS. Both white and African-American teens knew more than Latino youth. African-American and Latino adolescents were twice as likely as white adolescents to have misconceptions about casual transmission. African-American and Latino youth in this sample felt they were at greater risk than white respondents.[262]

By contrast, a study conducted in New York City in 1988 found that more than two-thirds of a sample of African-American and Hispanic teens had accurate information about HIV transmission. Unlike previous findings, this study revealed no difference between African Americans and Hispanics in knowledge. However, as shown in previous research, most of these adolescents harbored misconceptions about risk reduction (e.g., only 34% believed that abstinence reduced risk and 79% thought that oral contraceptives provided some protection from AIDS).[263]

Extremely low levels of knowledge about HIV infection and AIDS have been found in African-American female adolescents ages 13-15. In one study, only 30% of these young teens "passed" a test of AIDS knowledge by obtaining a score of 75% correct.[264] In another sample, even though female African-American and Hispanic adolescents were more likely to believe that condoms are a good way to decrease risk of HIV, they were less likely than males to insist on condom use.[265]

Noting the increasing incidence of AIDS in minority groups, Congress directed the Department of Health and Human Services to conduct a study of prevention programs targeting minority populations. The Health Omnibus Programs Extension of 1988 (Section 251) included a request that the Office of Minority Health study minority knowledge, attitudes, and beliefs regarding AIDS transmission and risk, and examine the effectiveness of AIDS prevention programs for minorities.[266] However, the data base used for the DHHS analysis (the National Health Interview Survey), includes only persons over the age of 18. Despite high levels of general knowledge about AIDS in all racial ethnic groups, whites have shown a greater knowledge of risk factors than other minority groups, and more knowledge of effective prevention strategies than African Americans.[267]

Socioeconomic and Cultural Factors Play Strong Roles in Success of Prevention/Intervention Strategies

The socioeconomic and cultural characteristics of racial and ethnic minority populations differ significantly from those of nonminority populations. Minority populations have experienced higher rates of poverty and unemployment and lower levels of education. Substantial percentages of minority populations live in inner cities, where they are more likely to experience substandard housing, crime, and other environmental hazards.[268]

Because poverty is also often associated with an inadequate social-support network, poor nutrition, and diminished access to health care, children growing up in poor or near-poor families probably confront more risks and benefit from fewer protections and supports than their more advantaged peers.[269] Like all behavior, AIDS risk-related behavior is tied to other facets of people's lives, and change in one realm can affect others.[270]

Psychosocial barriers to behavioral change characteristic of those in extreme poverty can include limited self-efficacy, low self-esteem, perceived peer group disapproval, or beliefs about lack of the control of the future.[271] Potentially compensating community strengths are described by Friedman, et al.:

> Minorities are constantly developing resources and dynamics of their own that aid their individual and collective struggles for survival, dignity, and happiness. These involve developing grapevines to carry information, networks to help each other out, and even formal organizations to formulate and achieve specific goals.[272]

Working through existing community entities is likely to be the most effective way to affect counterproductive community values and beliefs. Through them, HIV prevention/education programs can build on community strengths which may be neither recognized nor fully understood by outsiders. Consequently, key components of the community must be involved in both planning and carrying out the prevention strategy. The objective is to mobilize communities to utilize, or, if necessary, rebuild their social networks in order to stimulate and support sustained behavioral changes among their members.[273]

Diverse Minority Population Requires a Variety of Targeted HIV Interventions

The nation's ethnic and cultural diversity, apparent in language, cultural practices, beliefs about illness, and health-seeking behavior, requires the development of culturally appropriate HIV/AIDS information and education.[274] Although some of these cultural elements constitute barriers to HIV prevention that must be overcome, HIV prevention can build on other beliefs and practices that promote health, and should identify and respect cultural elements that do not threaten health.[275]

Similarities among cultures can suggest strategies for effective communication and education.[276] For example, one study found that among Asian and Pacific Islander cultures, family and community are vital parts of the lives of youths and the needs of the nuclear or extended family almost always supercede the needs of the individual.[277] Thus,..."for Asian-American adolescents, services that gain family involvement, use supportive family networks, and promote family decision-making are believed likely to be more effective, although there have been no tests of this model."[278]

However, when designing a program for the Asian and Pacific Islander communities, planners must take into account the diversity of these populations which include at least 43 different Asian and Pacific Islander groups from more than 40 countries and territories, and who speak more than 100 different languages and dialects. Materials and messages should be tested with local groups for acceptability and effectiveness.[279]

Latino communities in the United States exhibit heterogeneity despite a common language. Nuances of language or tradition can affect basic credibility and ultimate effectiveness. For example, in many Spanish speaking communities, "jeringa" means injecting equipment.[280] In Puerto Rico, however, "jeringa" means "don't bother me"; using this word may mean that a key prevention message would be incomprehensible to the segment of the Hispanic community with the highest rate of AIDS.[281]

Jose Duran, Executive Director of the Hispanic Office of Planning and Evaluation, Inc. (HOPE), testified at a Select Committee hearing that an AIDS intervention with Latino youth should be community-based, involve community outreach, present factual and explicit information, be bilingual, utilize peer leaders, and involve parents as well as adolescents. He also suggested use of focus groups to explore levels of acceptance of prevention messages in various forms.[282]

African-American communities have been most disproportionately affected by the HIV epidemic, but few have marshalled community resources to confront it.[283] A myriad of other, more immediately visible problems (including poverty, unemployment, racism, drugs, lower levels of education, and poor overall health), and distrust of the motives of the majority culture in imposing involvement,[(s)] prevent more immediate response to the threat of HIV infection.[285] Efforts to resolve these larger problems are crucial to the success of HIV interventions.[286]

Involving African-American people with AIDS in educational efforts can help overcome denial of the AIDS threat in African-American communities.[287] Some have also suggested that culture-specific barriers to sexual negotiation be taken into account in program planning.[288] The message should reach community members wherever they usually congregate, and should be a part of efforts to change the health-delivery system

---

(s) A recent study by Thomas and Crouse-Quinn describes the Tuskegee Syphilis study, led by the Public Health Service, which was the longest known nontherapeutic experiment on human beings in medical history.

The Tuskegee study tracked the results of deliberately untreated syphilis among African-American males over a 40 year period (1932 to 1972). Participants were never told that they were infected with a treatable disease, nor were they told that the disease could be transmitted sexually and from a mother to her fetus.

According to Thomas and Crouse-Quinn, strategies used to recruit and retain participants for this study were very similar to those being advocated for HIV/AIDS prevention programs in African-American communities today, including: extensive collaboration of community-based and grass-roots organizations, local churches, public schools, and the use of local African-American nurses and personnel.

The authors note: "Almost 60 years after the Tuskegee study began, there remains a trail of distrust and suspicion that hampers HIV education efforts in black communities."[284]

needs of the African-American family. To reach teens, prevention workers should target peer networks, so that protective attitudes will be reinforced over time. Verbal and nonverbal language that is "part of the cultural lexicon" should be a powerful tool for altering beliefs and behaviors in health-promoting directions.[289] According to Mays and Cochran, for African-Americans:

> ...[positive], ethnically-based values of cooperation and unity may be more powerful motivators of behavior change than strict appeals to individualistic action, such as "protect yourself." Successful civil rights activists, such as Martin Luther King, Jr., mobilized the Black community by calls for unity and faith in a vision for collective freedom.[290]

For Native Americans, "the realities of Indian life have been obscured due to centuries of multilayered stereotypes which continue to confound understanding and communication."[291] Like Hispanic and Asian Americans, Native Americans are not one homogeneous group. Numbering approximately two million,[292] Native Americans come from many nations or tribes, each with its own cultural heritage.[293]

The misconception that all Native Americans live on reservations contributes to the lack of visibility of the majority of Native Americans who live in cities or in non-reservation rural settings. This invisibility leads to problems with HIV seroprevalence data, AIDS case surveillance, and resource allocation.[294]

Although the problem of AIDS in Native American groups has not received much attention, it cannot be discounted. One recent study found that nearly half of rural Native American students worry a great deal about becoming infected with HIV. AIDS was among the top five worries for both males and females in grades 7-12.[295] As will be discussed further in another part of this chapter, abuse appears to play a strong role in increased sexual risk taking among Native American students. This study found that 49% of youth who reported having been physically abused have had intercourse, compared with 28% of those who had not been abused. The same pattern holds for youth who had been sexually abused. Fifty percent of sexually abused youth were sexually active compared with 29% of those who had not been physically abused.[296] Finally, as in other minority communities, growing numbers of AIDS cases among adult Native Americans may predict an increasing impact on youth.

Research On the Effectiveness of Prevention Programs For Minority Youth is Needed, Cultural Competence is Necessary, but Probably Insufficient to Guard the Health of Minority Youth in High-risk Situations

Comprehensive prevention programs, including access to health care, are key in reducing the risk of HIV infection, but they will have little impact on minority youth if they are insensitive to linguistic, social and cultural realities. Furthermore, it should be recognized that the adoption of health-promoting behaviors and attitudes can affect other areas of life,[297] resulting in economic and/or personal losses for individuals.[298]

Additional research is needed to address the issues involved in developing culturally sensitive prevention programs. Due to limited funding and the relative unavailability of trained minority researchers, there is a lack of data on minorities that could be useful in developing AIDS prevention strategies for minority teens.[299] The need for direction will not be met in the near future: when the Office of Minority Health studied the effectiveness of AIDS prevention programs for minorities of any age group, fewer than four of the 90 Public Health Service-funded projects examined were found to incorporate stringent evaluation design criteria in plans for future assessment.[300]

While it is critically important for services to be shaped by the cultural context of behavior that jeopardizes health, AIDS educators must also realize that cultural sensitivity alone does not guarantee behavior change in youth at highest risk. Beyond their membership in racial or ethnic minority groups, adolescents are individuals, and are most likely to respond to preventive efforts that address their individual needs and circumstances.[301] While this is a resource-intensive approach, the health of the minority adolescent community is at stake, and the growth rate of AIDS among minorities suggests that time is running out.[302]

G. INTERVENTIONS FOR HEMOPHILIAC YOUTH

Risk of Infection from Contaminated Blood Products Significantly Decreased, Services and Prevention Still Needed

More than 1,700 cases of AIDS have been identified in adults and adolescents with hemophilia and other coagulative blood disorders. Because hemophilia is a sex-linked genetic disease, many hemophiliacs are male. By the end of 1991, 242 adolescents ages 13-19 who had been diagnosed with AIDS had hemophilia or coagulation disorder.[303] (See Chapter I)

While more than half of the hemophiliacs in the United States are thought to be HIV positive as a function of receiving contaminated blood and blood products in the past,[304] few new cases due to contaminated blood have been documented in recent years. In 1985, a test was developed to screen blood for HIV antibodies, and current estimates of infection due to receipt of blood range from one in 40,000 to one in 153,000 units transfused.[305]

Sexual partners and children of HIV-infected hemophiliacs, however, continue to be at high risk of infection. In 1990, CDC provided $3 million to the Hemophilia Behavioral Intervention Evaluation Projects (conducted predominantly at federally-funded Hemophilia Treatment Centers [HTCs]) to assess strategies for preventing sexual and perinatal transmission in this population. Eleven of the sites involved in this project will include adolescents in their study groups,[306] but little is known at present about the effectiveness of behavioral risk-reduction among hemophiliac youth.[307]

In many cases, when hemophiliac children were tested for antibodies prior to adolescence, their parents were told of their status, but the youth themselves were not. Some of these individuals have become sexually active without knowing that they are infected with HIV.[308]

Even when individuals know their HIV status, there appear to be formidable psychological barriers to prevention efforts. This is evidenced by the finding that, despite high general knowledge about AIDS and how to prevent it among hemophiliacs, one study found that less than one-third of sexually-active hemophiliac males consistently use condoms.[309]

HIV-infected hemophiliac teens must struggle not only with the same psychosocial developmental challenges all teens face (e.g., management of an emerging sexuality), but also with unique pressures, including a constant awareness of serious health threats.[310] Thus, they are likely to require specialized medical management and psychosocial support.[311]

Partly as a result of the advocacy of the National Coordinating Committee (composed of Health Resources and Services Administration, Centers for Disease Control and the National Hemophilia Foundation), Federal efforts on behalf of hemophiliacs have included risk-reduction curriculum development, a grant program for psychosocial support services, and outreach to minority persons with hemophilia who may not be currently served by HTCs.[312] In addition, compared with other HIV-infected adolescents, a greater proportion of hemophiliac youth have been included in NIH clinical trials for new HIV/AIDS drugs. (See Chapter V for further discussion of these issues.)

The levels of medical and psychosocial services that are likely to be required by HIV-infected hemophiliac youth are potentially overwhelming to the resources of HTCs. An assessment is underway to determine the feasibility of integrating the comprehensive care services provided by the HTCs with the services of HIV-related health care agencies.[313]

Existing services are inadequate to meet the needs of HIV-infected adolescents, with or without complicating medical conditions such as hemophilia.[314] The Institute of Medicine recommended employing three basic strategies to address the service needs of HIV-infected youth: (1) expand existing services for other adolescent health problems to include HIV infection and AIDS; (2) expand adult HIV and AIDS programs to include adolescents; and (3) develop new programs specifically designed to treat HIV-infected teens. Not until the broader health care system serves the needs of all infected adolescents will adequate treatment for HIV-infected hemophiliac youth begin to be assured.[315]

H. CONSIDERATIONS FOR SERVING YOUTH WHO HAVE BEEN SEXUALLY ABUSED

While national statistics remain incomplete, available data show that child abuse reports have increased steadily over the last 10 years.[316] Estimates of the prevalence of sexual abuse vary depending on the definitions used. In 1990 alone, there were over 2,500,000 reports of maltreatment; 15% were reports of sexual abuse.[317] As is the case with child physical abuse, experts believe that child sexual abuse is vastly under-reported.[318] Conservatively, an estimated one in four females and one in six males are sexually assaulted before age 18.[319]

The relationship between childhood sexual abuse and risk of HIV infection is largely unexplored. It is impossible to determine how many children have been infected with HIV as a result of abuse.[320] One recent study of 96 HIV-infected children (ages 17 and younger) who were treated at Duke University between 1987 and 1989, confirmed that 14 (eight females and three males) had been sexually abused. Four of these children acquired HIV infection as a result of sexual abuse. For six others, abuse was a possible source of transmission.[321]

Research has begun to explore the link between child sexual abuse and subsequent high-risk behaviors. Studies have reported correlations between childhood sexual assault and behaviors that put adolescents and adults at high risk of HIV infection, such as sex with multiple partners, unprotected sex, and drug and alcohol use.[(t)]

(t) It is important to note that studies cited in this section indicate a correlational relationship between child sexual abuse and increased sexual and drug related risk taking, rather than a causal one. As noted by Louise Silvern, Associate Professor at the University of Colorado:

> The relationships between child abuse and such adult events may or may not indicate that abuse induces "risky" behavior....Moreover our results suggest that the relationship between child abuse and adult dangers are not specifically

A history of sexual abuse is only one factor among many that may predict subsequent risk-taking behavior.[322] However, adolescents who have been sexually abused have recently been identified as a population that should be targeted for HIV transmission.[323]

History of Childhood Sexual Abuse Correlated with Risky Sexual Behavior

A recent study of heterosexually active young adults in southeastern New England found increased sexual risk-taking among persons who reported a history of early sexual abuse. Compared with individuals who did not report a history of sexual abuse, abuse survivors were four times more likely to be working as prostitutes, twice as likely to report multiple sexual partners within a given year, and 40% more likely to report a sexual encounter with someone they did not know. Women who reported being sexually assaulted during childhood were almost three times more likely to become pregnant before age 18. Survivors of sexual abuse were only slightly more likely to report a history of STDs or to have serologic evidence of HIV infection. However, "men who reported early sexual abuse had a two-fold increase in prevalence of HIV infection relative to unabused men."[324]

Other studies indicate similar correlations between childhood abuse and high-risk behavior that might lead to HIV infection. A recent study of 535 young women who had become pregnant as adolescents found that two-thirds had been sexually abused (62% before first pregnancy). More than half (55%) had been molested, 44% had been raped, and 42% had been victims of attempted rape. Compared with young women who also became pregnant as adolescents but who had not been abused, sexually victimized females began intercourse at an earlier age (13.2 vs. 14.5), were more likely to have used alcohol or other drugs

---

mediated by their sexual nature....My concern about prematurely interpreting these data is that they not be used to futher stigmatize abused children or to encourage blaming adult victims by assuming that they have contributed to their ill-fate. (Personal Communication, July 23, 1991.)

during first intercourse (30% vs. 12%) and less likely to practice contraception at first intercourse (19% vs. 23%).[325]

A 1990 study of 600 students at an urban public high school found that students with a history of sexual abuse were more likely to engage in risk-taking, self-destructive behaviors. Students who had experienced sexual abuse were three and one-half times more likely to be sexually active as students who reported no history of sexual abuse.[326] Other studies found that many survivors of childhood sexual abuse report later sexual difficulties and multiple sexual partners.[327]

Correlations Also Evident Between Childhood Sexual Abuse and Increased Alcohol and Other Drug Use

Several researchers have observed relationships between sexual abuse and drug and alcohol use among adolescents. A 1989 study of 1,824 adolescents who received substance abuse treatment found that both male and female sexual abuse victims were more likely to have used a wider array of drugs than were their non-abused treatment counterparts. Nearly six in ten adolescents in the abused group used drugs (not including alcohol and marijuana) compared with four in ten adolescents in the control group.[328]

Other studies confirm these findings; youth who reported abuse were more likely to report regular cocaine and stimulant use and greater frequencies of alcohol and drug use. Abused youth also begin using alcohol and drugs at an earlier age than other adolescents.[329]

While researchers agree that victims of sexual abuse are generally at greater risk for alcohol and drug use, some investigators caution that our knowledge of this phenomenon is quite limited. Further research is needed to more clearly identify this relationship.[330]

Dynamics of Relationship Between Child Sexual Abuse and Adolescent HIV Largely Unexplored

While researchers have documented an association between

dynamics of this relationship remain unexplored. Similarly, little is known about the co-occurrence of problem behaviors.[331]

Research has begun to suggest that protective factors, including the youth's intelligence, temperament, cognitive appraisal of events, coping skills, support from a significant person, and positive placement experiences in foster care, may serve to buffer the effects of childhood victimization and help to mitigate later adolescent problem behaviors. It is essential to protect children from abuse in the first place, and further effort also should be directed at preventing the development of dysfunctional outcomes in adolescence and beyond.[332]

Endnotes

1 Kinsey, A., et al. "Sexual Behavior in the Human Male." 1948; Kinsey, A., et al. "Sexual Behavior in the Human Female." 1953. (Cited by U.S. Department of Health and Human Services [DHHS]. Report of the Secretary's Task Force on Youth Suicide - Vol. 3. "Gay Male and Lesbian Youth Suicide." Gibson, P. 1989.)

2 Kinsey, A., et al. 1948 and 1953. op cit.; Zenilman, J. "Sexually Transmitted Diseases in Homosexual Adolescents." Journal of Adolescent Health Care. Vol. 9. No. 2. March 1988.

3 Turner, C.F., et al. (eds.) National Research Council. AIDS: Sexual Behavior and Intravenous Drug Use. Washington, D.C.: National Academy Press. 1989.

4 Institute of Medicine. Report of a Study: The AIDS Research Program of the National Institutes of Health. Washington, D.C.: National Academy Press. 1991.

5 Turner, C.F., et al. (eds.) 1989. op cit.

6 Miller, H.G., et al. (eds.) AIDS: The Second Decade. Washington, D.C.: National Academy Press. 1990; American Academy of Pediatrics, Committee on Adolescence. "Homosexuality and Adolescence." Pediatrics. 1983; Cates, J.A. "Adolescent Sexuality: Gay and Lesbian Issues." Child Welfare. Journal of the Child Welfare League of American, Inc. Vol. LXVI. No. 4. July/August 1987.

7 Remafedi, G.J. "Preventing the Sexual Transmission of AIDS During Adolescence." Journal of Adolescent Health Care. Vol. 9. No. 2. March 1988.

8 U.S. Department of Health and Human Services, Centers for Disease Control (CDC). "HIV/AIDS Surveillance, Year End Edition, U.S. Cases Reported through December 1991." January 1992.

9 Turner, C.F., et al. (eds.) 1989. op cit.

10 Zenilman, J. 1988. op cit.; Stall, R., et al. "Behavioral Risk Reduction for HIV Infection Among Gay and Bisexual Men: A Review of Results From Across the United States." American Psychologist. Vol. 43. No. 11. 1988.

11 Stall, R., et al. 1988. op cit; Miller, H.G., et al. (eds.) 1990. op cit.

12 Zenilman, J. 1989. op cit.; Stall, R., et al. 1988. op cit.

13 Gardner, W. "Adolescents and AIDS: Epidemiology and Prevention." Testimony at hearing, The Risky Business of Adolescence: How To Help Teens Stay Safe. Select Committee on Children, Youth, and Families. U.S. House of Representatives. Washington, D.C. June 17, 1991; Miller, H.G., et al. (eds.) 1990. op cit.

14 Miller, H.G., et al. (eds.) 1990. op cit.

15 Feldman, D. "Gay Youth and AIDS." Journal of Homosexuality. Vol. 17. Nos. 1 and 2. 1989; "The Young Men's Survey: Principle Findings and Results, A Presentation to the San Francisco Health Commission." June 1991; Remafedi, G.J. "Fundamental Issues in the Care of Homosexual Youth." Medical Clinics of North America. Vol. 74. No. 5. September 1990.

16 "The Young Men's Survey: Principle Findings and Results, A Presentation to the San Francisco Health Commission." June 1991.

17 Owen, W.F., Jr. "Medical Problems of the Homosexual Adolescent." Journal of Adolescent Health Care. Vol. 6. No. 4. 1985.

18 Owen, W.F., Jr. 1985. op cit.

19 Chu, S.Y., et al. "Epidemiology of Reported Cases of AIDS in Lesbian, United States 1980-89." American Journal of Public Health. Vol. 80. No. 11. 1990.

20 Rotheram-Borus, M.J., et al. "The Relationship of Knowledge and Attitudes Towards AIDS to Safe Sex Practices Among Runaway and Gay Adolescents." HIV Center for Clinical and Behavioral Studies, Columbia University, NY. Unpublished.

21 Remafedi, G.J. "Adolescent Homosexuality: Psychosocial and Medical Implications." Pediatrics. Vol. 79. 1987. (Cited by Remafedi, G.J. 1988. op cit.)

22 Zenilman, J. 1988. op cit.

23 Remafedi, G.J. 1987. op cit.

24 Miller, H.G., et al. (eds.) 1990. op cit.; Remafedi, G.J. September 1990. op cit.; Feldman, D. 1989. op cit; Zenilman, J. 1988. op cit.

25 American Academy of Pediatrics. 1983. op cit.; Troiden, R.R. "Homosexual Identity Development." Journal of Adolescent Health Care. Vol. 9. No. 2. March 1988.

26 Remafedi, G.J. "The Care of Gay and Lesbian Youth." Proceedings from the 1989 Adolescent Health Coordinators Conference. Denver, CO. August 1989. National Center for Education in Maternal and Child Health: Washington, D.C.

27 Hunter, J. and Schaecher, R. "Lesbian and Gay Youth." Rotheram-Borus, M.J., et al. (eds.) Planning to Live: Suicide Prevention Among Teens in Community Settings. Tulsa, Oklahoma: University of Oklahoma Press. 1990.

28 American Academy of Pediatrics. 1983. op cit.

29 Remafedi, G.J. 1988. op cit.

30 Cates, J.A. 1987. op cit.

31 Martin, A.D. and Hetrick, E.S. "Designing an AIDS Risk Reduction Program for Gay Teenagers: Problems and Proposed Solutions." Ostrow, D.G. (ed.) Behavioral Control of AIDS. New York, NY: Irvington Publishers, Inc. 1987; Remafedi, G.J. 1988. op cit.

32 Hunter, J. and Schaecher, R. "Stresses on Lesbian and Gay Adolescents in Schools." Social Work in Education. Vol. 9. No. 3. Spring 1987.

33 U.S. General Accounting Office (GAO). AIDS Education: Public School Programs Require More Student Information and Teacher Training. GAO/HRD-90-103. Report to the Chairman, Committee on Governmental Affairs, U.S. Senate. May 1990.

34 GAO. GAO/HRD-90-103. May 1990. op cit.; Martin, A.D. "Testimony to the President's Commission on the HIV Epidemic." Washington, D.C. May 17, 1988.

35 McManus, M.C. "Serving Lesbian and Gay Youth." Focal Point: The Bulletin of the Research and Training Center on Family Support and Children's Mental Health. Vol. 5. No. 2. Spring/Summer 1991.

36 McManus, M.C. 1991. op cit.

37 Martin, A.D. 1988. op cit.

38 Hetrick, E.S. and Martin, A.D. "Developmental Issues and Their Resolution for Gay and Lesbian Adolescents." Journal of Homosexuality. 1987.

39 Gardner, W. 1991. op cit.

40 Dennis, D.I. and Harlow, R.E. "Gay Youth and the Right to Education." Yale Law and Policy Review. Vol. IV. No. 2. Spring/Summer 1986.

41 National Gay Task Force. "Anti-Gay/Lesbian Victimization." New York. 1984. (Cited by DHHS. 1989. op cit.)

42 Remafedi, G.J. September 1990. op cit; DHHS. 1989. op cit.

43 Hunter, J. "Violence Against Lesbian and Gay Youths." 1990. In Press.

44 DHHS. 1989. op cit.

45 "Cut Down as They Grow Up: AIDS Stalks Gay Teenagers." The New York Times. New York, N.Y. December 13, 1990.

46 DHHS. 1989. op cit.

47 Remafedi, G.J. September 1990. op cit.

48 Hunter, J. and Schaecher, R. 1987. op cit.

49 DHHS. 1989. op cit.

50 DHHS. National Center for Health Statistics. "Monthly Vital Statistics Report." Vol. 39. No. 12. April 1991.

51 DHHS. 1989. op cit.

52 Remafedi, G.J, et al. "Risk Factors for Attempted Suicide in Gay and Bisexual Youth." Pediatrics. Vol. 87. No. 6. 1991. (Cited by Farrow, J.A. "Gay and Lesbian Youth Suicide." Focal Point: The Bulletin of the Research and Training Center on Family Support and Children's Mental Health. Vol 5. No. 2. Spring/Summer 1991.)

53 Remafedi, G.J. 1988. op cit.

54 Lehman, M.P. Human Rights Campaign Fund. Written testimony submitted for hearing, The Risky Business of Adolescence: How To Help Teens Stay Safe. Select Committee on Children, Youth, and Families. U.S. House of Representatives. Washington, D.C., June 18, 1991; Gardner, W. 1991. op cit.; McManus, M.C. 1991. op cit.; Remafedi, G.J. 1991. op cit.

55 Human Rights Campaign Fund. 1991. op cit.

56 McManus, M.C. 1991. op cit.; Human Rights Campaign Fund. 1991. op cit.; DHHS. 1989. op cit.

57 Martin, A.D. 1988. op cit.; McManus, M.C. 1991. op cit.; Human Rights Campaign Fund. 1991. op cit.; DHHS. 1989. op cit.

58 GAO. GAO/HRD-70-103. 1990. op cit.; Kolbe, L.J., Personal Communication. August 1991; Select Committee key informant interviews, personal communication, August 1991; Lehman, M.P. Human Rights Campaign Fund. Personal Communication. March 1992.

59 Hunter, J. "Intervention Model: Working With Gay and Lesbian Youth at Risk for HIV Infection." Meeting Abstract. International Conference on AIDS. June 1989; Remafedi, G.J. September 1990. op cit.; Human Rights Campaign Fund. 1991. op cit.

60 Rotheram-Borus, M.J., et al. "Sexual and Substance Abuse Behaviors Among Homosexual and Bisexual Male Adolescents in New York City." In Press.

61 Remafedi, G.J. "HIV Risk and Prevention Among Gay/Bisexual Youth." Abstract. Journal of Adolescent Health. Vol. 12. No. 2. March 1990.

62 Remafedi, G.J. March 1990. op cit.; Remafedi, G.J. "The University of Minnesota Youth and AIDS Project, Executive Summary: Client Data." Unpublished.

63 Remafedi, G.J. March 1990. op cit.

64 Remafedi, G.J. Unpublished. op cit.

65 U.S. Department of Justice. Office of Juvenile Justice and Delinquency Prevention (OJJDP). Missing, Abducted, Runaway, and Thrownaway Children in America - Executive Summary. May 1990.

66 GAO. AIDS Education: Programs for Out-of-School Youth Slowly Evolving. GAO/HRD-90-111. May 1990.

67 Robertson, M. "Homeless Youth: An Overview of the Literature." Paper delivered at conference on Homeless Children and Youth. Coping with a National Tragedy. Washington, D.C. May 1989. (Cited by Athey, J.L. "HIV Infection and Homeless Adolescents." Child Welfare. Vol. LXX. No. 5. September-October 1991.)

68 Finkelhor, D., et al. Missing, Abducted, Runaway, and Thrownaway Children in America. Washington, D.C.: U.S. Department of Justice. 1990. (Cited by Athey, J.L. 1991. op cit.)

69 Stricof, R.L., et al. "HIV Seroprevalence in a Facility for Runaway and Homeless Adolescents." American Journal of Public Health. Vol. 50, 81 Supplement. May 1991. (Cited by Athey, J.L. 1991. op cit.)

70 Daley, S. "New York City Street Youth: Living in the Shadow of AIDS." The New York Times. New York, N.Y. November 14, 1988. (Cited by Rotheram-Borus, M.J. and Koopman, S. "Research on AIDS Prevention among Runaways: The State of the Art and Recommendations for the Future." Paper presented at the National Institute of Child Health and Human Development Technical Review and Research Planning Meeting on Adolescents and HIV Infection. January 12, 1989.)

71 Office of the Inspector General. January 1991. op cit.

72 Rotheram-Borus, M.J., et al. "Homeless Youths and HIV Infection." American Psychologist. Vol. 46. No. 11. November 1991.

73 Rotheram-Borus, M.J. Testimony at hearing, The Risky Business of Adolescence: How to Help Teens Stay Safe. Select Committee on Children, Youth and Families. U.S. House of Representatives. Washington, D.C. June 17, 1991.

74 GAO. Homelessness: Homeless and Runaway Youth Receiving Services at Federally Funded Shelters. HRD-90-45. Report to The Honorable Paul Simon. U.S. Senate. Washington D.C.: GAO. December 1989.

75 Gammon, M. (Cited by Hermann, R.C. "Center Provides Approach to Major Social Ill: Homeless Urban Runaways, 'Throwaways.'" Journal of the American Medical Association. Vol. 260. No. 3. July 15, 1988.)

76 The Stanford Center for the Study of Families, Children and Youth. The Stanford Studies of Homeless Families, Children and Youth. Stanford, CA. November 18, 1991.

77 Browne, A., and Finkelhor, D. "Initial and Long-term Effects: A Review of the Research." Finkelhor, D. (ed.) Sourcebook on Child Sexual Abuse. Beverly Hills, CA: Sage. 1986. (Cited by Athey, J.L. 1991. op cit.)

78 Child and Adolescent Service System Program (CASSP). On Their Own: Runaway and Homeless Youth and Programs That Serve Them. Washington, D.C. June 1991.

79 Seattle Department of Human Resources. Report on Gay and Lesbian Youth in Seattle. Seattle, WA: Commission on Children and Youth. 1988. (Cited by Athey, J.L. 1991. op cit.)

80 Humm, A. New York, NY. Hetrick-Martin Institute. December 14, 1989. Personal Communication with The Center for Population Options (CPO) as reported in Out of the Shadows: Building an Agenda and Strategies for Preventing HIV/AIDS in Street and Homeless Youth. 1990.

81 The Council on Scientific Affairs. American Medical Association. "Health Care Needs of Homeless and Runaway Youth." Journal of The American Medical Association. Vol. 262. No. 10. (Cited by CPO. 1990. op cit.)

82 Manov, A. and Lowther, L. "A Health Care Approach for Hard-to-reach Adolescent Runaways." Nurse Clinicians of North America. Vol. 18. 1983 (Cited by Athey. 1991. op cit.); "Teen Prostitutes." The Washington Post. Washington, D.C. December 6, 1988.

83 Coburn, J.H.S. Testimony at hearing, Aids Education for School-Aged Youth. Committee on Governmental Affairs. U.S. Senate. Washington, D.C. May 3, 1990.

84 The Washington Post. 1988. op cit.

85 Athey, J.L. 1991. op cit.

86 Yates, G.L., et al. "A Risk Profile Comparison of Runaway and Non-runaway Youth." The American Journal of Public Health. Vol. 78. No. 37. July 1988.

87 GAO. 1989. op cit.

88 Rotheram-Borus, M.J., et al. "Reducing HIV Sexual Risk Behaviors Among Runaway Adolescents." The Journal of the American Medical Association. Vol. 266. No. 9. September 4, 1991.

89 Wright, J.D. "Poverty, Homelessness, Health, Nutrition, and Children." Paper delivered at a conference on Homeless Children and Youth. Coping with A National Tragedy. Washington, D.C. May 1988.

90 Yates, G.L., et al. 1988. op cit.

91 Kelly, J.T. "Trauma: With the Example of San Francisco's Shelter Programs." Health Care of Homeless People. Brickner, L.K., et al. (eds.) 1985. (Cited by Athey, J.L. 1991. op cit.): Neinstein, L.S. and Stewart, D.C. Adolescent Health Care: A Practical Guide. Baltimore, Maryland. 1985. (Cited by Athey, J.L. 1991. op cit.)

92 Shaffer, D., and Caton, C.L.M. Runaway and Homeless Youth in New York City: A Report to the Ittleson Foundation. New York, NY: Division of Child Psychiatry. New York State Psychiatric Institute and Columbia University College of Physicians and Surgeons. 1984. (Cited by Athey, J.L. 1991. op cit.)

93 Able-Peterson, T. "The Most Forgotten Adolescents." Presentation at conference. Treatment of Adolescents with Alcohol, Drug Abuse, and Mental Health Problems. Alexandria, VA. October 1989. (Cited by Athey, J.L. 1991. op cit.)

94 Rotheram-Borus, M.J., et al. "Barriers to Successful AIDS Prevention Programs with Runaway Youth." Woodruff, J., et al. (eds.) Troubled Adolescents and HIV Infection: Issues in Prevention and Treatment. Washington, DC: Child and Adolescent Service System Program (CASSP). October 1989.

95 Coburn, J.H.S. 1990. op cit.

96 U.S. Congress. The Office of Technology Assessment (OTA). Adolescent Health - Volume II: Background and the Effectiveness of Selected Prevention and Treatment Services. Washington, D.C.: Government Printing Office. November 1991.

97 OTA. November 1991. op cit.

98 Hermann, R.C. 1988. op cit.

99 Coburn, J.H.S. 1990. op cit.

100 Rotheram-Borus, M.J., et al. 1989. op cit.; Shaffer, D., and Caton, C.L.M. 1984. op cit.

101 Rotheram-Borus, M.J., et al. 1989. op cit.

102 Office of the Inspector General. January 1991. op cit.

103 Athey, J.L. 1991. op cit.

104 Office of the Inspector General. January 1991. op cit.

105 OTA. November 1991. op cit.; GAO. 1989. op cit.; Rotheram-Borus, M.J., et al. November 1991. op cit.; English, A. "Runaway and Street Youth at Risk for Infection: Legal and Ethical Issues in Access to Care." July 1990. Used with permission.

106 Rotheram-Borus, M.J. June 1991. op cit.

107 GAO. 1989. op cit.

108 Rotheram-Borus, M.J. June 1991. op cit.

109 Rotheram-Borus, M.J., et al. September 1991. op cit.

110 Rotheram-Borus, M.J. June 1991. op cit.

111 Rotheram-Borus, M.J., et al. September 1991. op cit.

112 Coburn, J.H.S. 1990. op cit.

113 American Medical Association. Profiles of Adolescent Health: Adolescent Health Care; Use, Costs, and Problems of Access. Gans, J.E., et al. (eds.) 1991.

114 Rotheram-Borus, M.J., et al. November 1991. op cit.

115 Athey, J.L. 1991. op cit.

116 Council on Scientific Affairs, American Medical Association (AMA). "Health Status of Detained and Incarcerated Youths." Journal of the American Medical Association. Vol. 263. No. 7. February 1990.; National Commission on AIDS. Report: HIV Disease in Correctional Facilities. Washington, D.C. March 1991; OTA. November 1991. op cit.

117 National Commission on AIDS. March 1991. op cit.

118 U.S. Department of Justice. National Institute of Justice (NIJ). 1989 Update: AIDS in Correctional Facilities. May 1990.

119 Vlahov, D., et al. "Prevalence of Antibody to HIV-1 Among Entrants to U.S. Correctional Facilities." Journal of the American Medical Association. Vol. 265. No. 9. March 1991.

120 Vlahov, D., et al. 1991. op cit.

121 Miller, H.G., et al. (eds.) 1990. op cit.

122 Harrison, E. National Commission on Correctional Health Care (NCCHC). Testimony before the National Commission on AIDS. New York. August 17, 1990.

123 OJJDP. Juveniles Taken Into Custody: Fiscal Year 1990 Report. San Francisco, California: National Council on Crime and Delinquency. September 1991.

124 OJJDP. Public Juvenile Facilities: Children in Custody 1989. Washington, D.C.: OJJDP. January 1991.

125 U.S. Department of Justice. Bureau of Justice Statistics (BJS). Special Report: Survey of Youth in Custody, 1987. Washington, D.C.: BJS. September 1988.

126 Williams, Polly. Congressional Liaison to Mr. Sweet, (former) Administrator, OJJDP. February 4, 1992.

127 BJS. 1988. op cit.

128 BJS. 1988. op cit.

129 Marquis, D. NCCHC. Written testimony submitted for hearing, Risky Business of Adolescence: How To Help Teens Stay Safe. Select Committee on Children, Youth, and Families. U.S. House of Representatives. Washington, D.C. June 18, 1991.

130 Marquis, D. NCCHC. 1991. op cit.

131 Marquis, D. NCCHC. 1991. op cit.

132 DiClemente, R.J., et al. "Comparison of AIDS Knowledge, Attitudes, and Behaviors Among Incarcerated Adolescents and a Public School Sample in San Francisco." American Journal of Public Health. Vol. 81. No. 5. May 1991.

133 Nader, M.D., et al. "Comparison of Beliefs About AIDS Among Urban, Suburban, Incarcerated, and Gay Adolescents." Journal of Adolescent Health Care. Vol. 10. No. 5. 1989.

134 Hein, K., et al. "Age at First Intercourse Among Homeless Adolescent Females." Journal of Pediatrics. Vol. 93. (Cited by Miller, H.G., et. al. [eds.] 1991. op cit.)

135 Council on Scientific Affairs, American Medical Association. 1990. op cit.

136 Rolf, J., et al. "Issues in AIDS Prevention Among Juvenile Offenders." Woodruff, J.O., et al. (eds.) Troubled Adolescents and HIV Infection: Issues in Prevention and Treatment. Washington, D.C.: CASSP Technical Assistance Center. October 1989.

137 Baker, C.J. "HIV Infection and Policy Issues in Juvenile Correctional Facilities, Los Angeles County." Unpublished paper. Department of Health Services, Los Angeles County.

138 Key informant survey responses from Gary Shostak, M.P.H., Director of Health Services, Commonwealth of Massachusetts, Department of Youth Services. Personal Communication. 1991.

139 Council on Scientific Affairs, American Medical Association. 1990. op cit.

140 Lanier, M.M. and McCarthy, B.R. "AIDS Education and the Impact of AIDS Education in Juvenile Corrections." Criminal Justice and Behavior. Vol. 16. No. 4. December 1989.

141 Hammett, T. "AIDS in Correctional Facilities: Issues and Options, (3rd Edition)." NIJ. 1988. (Cited by Lanier, M.M. and McCarthy, B.R. 1989. op cit.

142 American Correctional Association. "Incidence of AIDS Among Juveniles in Corrections and Detention Facilities: AIDS Survey." Washington, D.C.: OJJDP. (Cited by Lanier, M.M. and McCarthy, B.R. 1989. op cit.)

143 NIJ. May 1990. op cit.

144 Hager, L. & Bibus, D. (in preparation) MOD Project Evaluation Summary: YouthCare, University of Washington School of Social Work.

145 Bazemore, G. "Youth Participation Strategies for the Juvenile Justice System: Obstacles and Opportunities." Future Choices, Empowerment Series. 1991.

146 NCCHC. "Policy Statement Regarding the Administrative Management of HIV in Corrections." Chicago, IL. Most recent revision, September 22, 1991.

147 NCCHC. Health Education Policies and Curricula for Incarcerated Youth: Trainer's Manual. Chicago, IL. 1991.

148 Marquis, D. NCCHC. 1991. op cit.

149 No Place to Call Home: Discarded Children in America. Select Committee on Children, Youth, and Families. Report 101-395. Washington, D.C.: U.S. Government Printing Office. 1990.

150 Assistant Secretary for Planning and Evaluation, DHHS. A Report on Infants and Children with HIV Infection in Foster Care. Washington, D.C. September 1990.

151 American Public Welfare Association (APWA). Interstate Compact on Adoption and Medical Assistance, Issue Brief: State Policies for Foster Care and Adoption for HIV-positive Children. No. IX. Washington, D.C.: APWA. November, 1989.

152 Polit, D.F., et al. "Sex, Contraception and Pregnancy among Adolescents in Foster Care." Family Planning Perspectives. Vol. 21. No. 5. 1989.

153 Polit, D.F., et al. 1989. op cit.

154 Rotheram-Borus, M.J., et al. 1989. op cit.

155 Joint Congressional hearing, Foster Care, Child Welfare, and Adoption Reforms. Committee on Ways and Means, Subcommittee on Public Assistance and Unemployment Compensation, and Select Committee on Children, Youth, and Families. U.S. House of Representatives. Washington, D.C. April 13, 1988.

156 Overview of Entitlement Programs: 1991 Green Book. A Report of the Committee on Ways and Means. U.S. House of Representatives. Washington, D.C. May 7, 1991.

157 Tatara, T. Characteristics of Children in Substitute and Adoptive Care: Statistical Summary of the VCIS National Child Welfare Data Base, FY82-FY88. Washington, D.C.: APWA. (in press)

158 Tatara, T. VCIS Research Notes. Vol. 3. Washington, D.C.: APWA. 1991.

159 Wulczyn, F.H. and George, R.M. "Foster Care in New York and Illinois: The Challenge of Rapid Change." Paper available from the second author at the Chapin Hall Center for Children, University of Chicago. 1991.

160 Euster, S.D., et al. "Life Skills Groups for Adolescent Foster Children." Child Welfare League of America. Vol. 63. No. 1. 1984.

161 Child Welfare League of America (CWLA). Too Young to Run. Washington, D.C.: CWLA. 1986; George, R.M. Personal Communication. Chapin Hall Center for Children, University of Chicago. 1991.

162 Jones, R., et al. "Adolescents with AIDS in Foster Care: A Case Report." Troubled Adolescents and HIV Infection: Issues in Prevention and Treatment. Washington, D.C.: CASSP Technical Assistance Center. 1989.

163 Jones, R., et al. 1989. op cit.

164 Annin, J.B., et al. CWLA. Personal Communication. September 3, 1991.

165 Grayson, M. Testimony at Joint Congressional hearing, Foster Care, Child Welfare, and Adoption Reforms. Committee on Ways and Means, Subcommittee on Public Assistance and Unemployment Compensation, and Select Committee on Children, Youth, and Families. U.S. House of Representatives. Washington, D.C. April 13, 1988.

166 OTA. Adolescent Health--Volume I: Summary and Policy Options. Washington, D.C.: U.S. Government Printing Office. April 1991.

167 Wells, E. "Child Welfare's Response to the Challenge of Serving Children with HIV." Courts, Health Science & The Law. Vol. 2. No. 1. Summer 1991. Georgetown University, Washington, D.C. 1991.

168 Tourse, P. and Gundersen, L. "Adopting and Fostering Children with AIDS: Policies in Progress." Children Today. May-June 1988.

169 APWA. "Foster Care Rates." W/Memo. Vol. 2. No. 4. 1990.

170 Annin, J.B. CWLA. Personal Communication. July 25, 1991.

171 Arizona Department of Economic Security. Acquired Immune Deficiency Syndrome (AIDS) Policy. March 1, 1990.

172 Wells, E. 1991. op cit.

[173] Wells, E., "State Policies for Foster Care and Adoption for HIV-Positive Children." Interstate Compact on Adoption and Medical Assistance Issue Brief. November, 1989.

[174] Wells, E. 1991. op cit.

[175] English, A. National Center for Youth Law. Personal Communication. March 1992.

[176] Wells, E. 1991. op cit.

[177] English, A. 1992. op cit.

[178] Wells, E. 1989. op cit.

[179] Polit, D.F., et al. "Sex Education and Family Planning Services for Adolescents in Foster Care." Family Planning Perspectives. Vol. 19. No. 18. 1987.

[180] Polit, D.F. 1987. op cit.

[181] Polit, D.F. 1987. op cit.

[182] Danziger, S., et al. Adolescent Pregnancy Prevention in Wisconsin--The Need for Comprehensive Policies. Madison, WI: Department of Health and Social Services. 1980.

[183] Polit, D.F. 1987. op cit.

[184] Morton, T.D. Adolescent Pregnancy and Child Welfare Services. National Child Welfare Leadership Center, University of North Carolina, Chapel Hill. 1984.

[185] Polit, D.F. 1987. op cit.

[186] Polit, D.F. 1987. op cit.

[187] Annin, J.B. CWLA. 1991. op cit.

[188] Hippler, M. "The Problems and Promise of Gay Youth." Advocate. No. 455. September 16, 1986.

[189] Berlin, J. "Long-term Placement at Huckleberry's." In: Reaching Troubled Youth: Runaways and Community Mental Health. Gordon, J.S. and Beyer, M. (eds.) DHHS (ADM) 81-955. 1981.

190 Allen, M., et al. Teens in Foster Care: Preventing Pregnancy and Building Self-Sufficiency. Washington, D.C.: Children's Defense Fund's Adolescent Pregnancy Prevention Clearinghouse. 1987.

191 Annin, J.B. CWLA. 1991. op cit.

192 Wild, P. CHAAT Program, Family and Children's Services of Chatanooga, Tennessee, Inc. Personal Communication. 1992.

193 McKee, A. National Foster Care Resource Center for Family, Group, and Residential Care, Eastern Michigan University, Ypsilanti, Michigan. Personal Communication. 1991.

194 The National Network of Runaway and Youth Services, Safe Choices Project. Safe Choices Guide: AIDS and HIV Policies and Prevention Programs for High-Risk Youth. National Resource Center for Youth Services, University of Oklahoma. 1990.

195 Pressma, D. and Emery, L.J. Report of the CWLA Task Force on Children and HIV Infection: Initial Guidelines. Washington, D.C.: CWLA. 1988; Ryan, C.M. and Emery, L.J. Meeting the Challenge of HIV Infection in Family Foster Care. Washington, D.C.: CWLA. 1991.

196 Spar, K. Child Welfare and Foster Care Reform: Issues for Congress. Congressional Research Service, Library of Congress. December 13, 1991.

197 Federal Programs Affecting Children and Their Families. A Report of the Select Committee on Children, Youth, and Families. U.S. House of Representatives. Washington, D.C. 1990.

198 Flavin, D.K. and Frances, R.J. "Risk Taking Behavior, Substance Abuse Disorders, and the Acquired Immunodeficiency Syndrome." Advances in Alcohol and Substance Abuse. Vol. 6. 1987.

199 Fullilove, R.E., et al. "Risk of Sexually Transmitted Disease Among Black Adolescent Crack Users in Oakland and San Francisco, California." Journal of The American Medical Association. Vol. 263. 1990.

200 CDC. January 1992. op cit.

201 CDC. January 1992. op cit.

202 Miller, H.G., et al. 1990. op cit.

203 Ginzburg, H.M. "Acquired Immune Deficiency Syndrome (AIDS) and Drug Abuse." Galea, R.P., et al. (eds.) *AIDS and IV Drug Abusers: A Current Perspective*. Owings Mills, MD: National Health Publishing., 1988.

204 U.S. Department of Health and Human Services. National Institute on Drug Abuse (NIDA). *National Household Survey on Drug Abuse: Population Estimates 1991*. ADM 91-1732. Rockville, MD: NIDA. 1991.

205 Holtzman, D., et al. "HIV Instruction, HIV Knowledge, and Drug Injection Among High School Students in the United States." *American Journal of Public Health*. Vol. 81. 1991.

206 NIDA. ADM 91-1732. 1991. op cit.

207 NIDA. *Drug Use among American High School Seniors, College Students and Young Adults, 1975-1990. Volume 1 High School Seniors*. ADM 91-1835. Rockville, MD: NIDA. 1991.

208 CDC. "Alcohol and Other Drug Use among High School Students -- United States, 1990." *MMWR*. Vol. 40. 1991.

209 Chaisson, R.E., et al. "Cocaine Use and HIV Infection in Intravenous Drug Users in San Francisco." *Journal of the American Medical Association*. Vol. 261. 1989.

210 Fullilove, R.E., et al. 1990. op cit.

211 Fullilove, R.E., et al. 1990. op cit.

212 NIDA. ADM 91-1835. 1991. op cit.

213 U.S. Department of Health and Human Services, Office of the Inspector General. *Youth and Alcohol: A National Survey*. June 1991.

214 Stall, R., et al. "Alcohol and Drug Use During Sexual Activity and Compliance with Safe Sex Guidelines for AIDS: The AIDS Behavioral Research Project." *Health Education Quarterly*. Vol. 13. 1986; Ensminger, M.E. "Adolescent Sexual Behavior as It Relates to Other Transition Behaviors in Youth." Hofferth, S.L. and Hayes, C.D. (eds.) *Risking the Future: Adolescent Sexuality,*

Pregnancy, and Childbearing. Washington, D.C.: National Academy Press. 1987.

215 Hingson, R.W., et al. "Beliefs About AIDS, Use of Alcohol and Unprotected Sex Among Massachusetts Adolescents." American Journal of Public Health. Vol. 80. 1990.

216 OTA. November 1991. op cit.

217 Morehouse, E. "The Student Assistance Program: An Alcohol and Drug Abuse Prevention Model." Aronowit, E. (ed.) Prevention Strategies for Mental Health. New York, N.Y.: Neale Watson Academic Publications. 1983.

218 OTA. November 1991. op cit.

219 OTA. November 1991. op cit.

220 OTA. November 1991. op cit.

221 NIDA. The Adolescent Assessment Referral System Manual. Rockville, MD: NIDA. 1991.

222 National Association of State Alcohol and Drug Abuse Directors (NASADAD). Treatment Works: The Tragic Cost of Undervaluing Treatment in the "Drug War". Washington, D.C.: NASADAD. 1990.

223 NASADAD. 1990. op cit.

224 OTA. November 1991. op cit.

225 Miller, H.G., et al. 1990. op cit.

226 Miller, H.G., et al. 1990. op cit.

227 Ginzberg, H.M. 1988. op cit.

228 OTA. November 1991. op cit.

229 National Academy of Sciences. Institute of Medicine, Division of Health Care Services, Committee for the Substance Abuse Coverage Study. Treating Drug Problems. Washington, D.C.: National Academy Press. 1990.

230 OTA. November 1991. op cit.

231 OTA. November 1991. op cit.

232 Hubbard, R., et al. Treatment Outcome Prospective Study (TOPS): Client Characteristics and Behaviors Before, During, and After Treatment. Chapel Hill, N.C.: University of North Carolina Press. 1984; Sells, S.B., and Simpson, D.D. "Evaluation of Treatment Outcome for Youths in the Drug Abuse Reporting Program: A Follow up Study." Beschner, C.C. (ed.) Youth Drug Abuse: Problems, Issues, and Treatments. Lexington, Massachusetts: Lexington Books. 1979.

233 Amini, R., et al. "A Controlled Study of Inpatient vs. Outpatient Treatment of Delinquent Drug Abuse Adolescents: One Year Results." Comprehensive Psychiatry. Vol. 23. 1982.

234 OTA. November 1991. op cit.

235 Public Law 101-226, Drug Free Schools and Communities Act Amendments of 1989. Sec. 1213.

236 GAO. Drug Abuse Prevention. Federal Efforts to Identify Exemplary Programs Need Stronger Design. Washington, D.C.: GAO. 1991.

237 20 U.S.C. 317, Sec. 3212; Olsen, L.K. American School Health Association. Personal Communication to Allen King, Division of Drug Free Schools and Communities. October 1990.

238 Goodstadt, M.S. Drug Education. National Institute of Justice Crime File Study. Washington, D.C. US Department of Justice. 1988.

239 GAO. 1991. op cit.

240 GAO. 1991. op cit.

241 National Association of State Boards of Education (NASBE) and Council of Chief State School Officers (CCSSO). AIDS, HIV, and School Health Education: State Policies and Programs 1990. 1991.

242 U.S. Department of Health and Human Services, Office of Substance Abuse Prevention (OSAP). Preventing HIV Infection Among Youth. Rockville, Maryland: DHHS. 1991.

[243] Dryfoos, J.G. Adolescents at Risk: Prevalence and Prevention. New York: Oxford University Press. 1990.

[244] OSAP. 1991. op cit.

[245] OSAP. 1991. op cit.

[246] OSAP. 1991. op cit.

[247] Tobler, N.S. "Meta-Analysis of 143 Adolescent Drug Prevention Programs: Qualitative Outcome Results of Program Participants Compared to A Control or Comparison Group." Journal of Drug Issues. Vol. 14. No. 4. 1986.

[248] Tobler, N.S. 1986. op cit.

[249] U.S. Department of Education and DHHS. Report to ?Congress and the White House on the Nature and Effectiveness of Federal, State, and Local Drug Prevention/Education Programs. Washington, D.C. 1987; Dryfoos, J.G. 1990. op cit.

[250] Pentz, M.A., et al. "A Comprehensive Community Approach to Adolescent Drug Abuse Prevention: Effects on Cardiovascular Disease Risk Behaviors." Annals of Medicine. Vol. 21. 1989.

[251] Wodraska, D. Testimony at Hearing. The Risky Business of Adolescence: How to Help Teens Stay Safe. Select Committee on Children, Youth, and Families. U.S. House of Representatives. Washington, D.C. June 17, 1991.

[252] Lee, D.A. and Fong, K. "HIV/AIDS and the Asian and Pacific Islander Community." SEICUS REPORT. Vol. 18. No. 3. 1990.

[253] CDC. Special Data Run. January 13, 1992.

[254] CDC. January 13, 1992. op cit.

[255] OTA. Adolescent Health -- Volume III: Cross Cutting Issues in the Delivery of Health and Related Services. Washington, D.C.: Government Printing Office. June 1991.

[256] Diclemente, R.J. "Epidemiology of AIDS, HIV Prevalence and HIV Incidence Among Adolescents." Journal of School Health. Used with permission. (in press)

257 Cates, W. "The Epidemiology and Control of Sexually Transmitted Diseases in Adolescents." Adolescent Medicine: State of the Art Reviews. Vol. 1. No. 3. October. Philadelphia, PA: Hanley & Belfus, Inc. (CDC reprint) 1990.

258 NIDA. National Household Survey on Drug Abuse: Population Estimates 1991. 1991.

259 DiClemente, R.J. "Determinants of Condom Use Among Junior High School Students in a Minority, Inner-City School District." Center for AIDS Prevention Studies, University of California-San Francisco. (in press)

260 Blum, R., et al. The State of Native American Youth Health. University of Minnesota. Minneapolis, MN. March 1992.

261 Blum, R., et al. 1992. op cit.

262 DiClemente R.J., et al. "Minorities and AIDS: Knowledge, Attitudes, and Misconceptions among Black and Latino Adolescents." American Journal of Public Health. Vol. 78. 1988.

263 Goodman, E. and Cohall, A.T. "AIDS and Adolescents: Knowledge, Attitudes, Beliefs, and Behaviors in a New York City Adolescent Minority Population." Pediatrics, Vol. 84. No. 1. 1989.

264 Jaffe, L.R., et al. "Anal Intercourse and Knowledge of Acquired Immunodeficiency Syndrome Among Minority-Group Female Adolescents." Journal of Pediatrics. Vol. 112. 1988.

265 Goodman, E. and Cohall, A.T. 1989. op cit.

266 Public Law 101-607, Health Omnibus Programs Extension of 1988. Sec. 251.

267 U.S. Department of Health and Human Services, Office of Minority Health. Report to Congress: Aids Knowledge and the Effectiveness of Aids Prevention Interventions in Minority Communities. Washington, D.C. 1990.

268 U.S. Department of Health and Human Services. Report on the Secretary's Task Force on Black and Minority Health. Washington, D.C. 1985.

269 OTA. June 1991. op cit.

270 Mays, V.M. and Cochran, S.D. "Issues in the Perception of AIDS Risk and Risk Reduction Activities by Black and Hispanic/Latina Women." American Psychologist. Vol. 43. No. 11. 1988; Winett, R.A. Information and Behavior: Systems of Influence. Hillsdale, NJ: Erlbaum. 1986.

271 Mays, V.M. and Cochran, S.D. 1988. op cit.

272 Friedman, S.R., et al. "The AIDS Epidemic among Blacks and Hispanics." The Milbank Quarterly. Vol. 65. No. 2. 1987.

273 Bowles, J. and Robinson, W. "PHS Grants for Minority Group HIV Infection Education and Prevention Efforts." Public Health Reports. Vol. 104. 1989.

274 Airhihenbuwa, C.O., et al. HIV/AIDS Education and Prevention among African-Americans: A Focus on Culture. Manuscript available from the author, Health Education Department, Pennsylvania State University, University Park, PA, 16802. (in press)

275 Airhihenbuwa, C.O. (in press) op cit.

276 Mays, V.M. and Cochran, S.D. 1988. op cit.

277 Mays, V.M. and Cochran, S.D. 1988. op cit.

278 OTA. June 1991. op cit.

279 Lee, D.A. and Fong K. 1990. op cit.

280 National Commission on AIDS. "HIV Disease in Hispanic Communities." Transcript of Conference Proceedings. Washington, D.C. March 1991.

281 National Commission on AIDS. 1991. op cit.

282 Duran, J. Testimony at hearing. The Risky Business of Adolescence: How to Help Teens Stay Safe. Select Committee on Children, Youth, and Families. U.S. House of Representatives. Washington, D.C. June 18, 1991.

283 Gasch, H., et al. "Shaping AIDS Education and Prevention Programs for African Americans Amidst Community Decline." Journal of Negro Education. Vol. 60. No. 1. 1991.

284 Thomas, S.B. and Crouse Quinn, S. "Public Health Then and Now - The Tuskegee Syphilis Study, 1932 to 1972: Implications for HIV Education and AIDS Risk Education Programs in the Black Community." American Journal of Public Health. Vol. 81. No. 11. November 1991.

285 National Commission on AIDS. March 1991. op cit.; Dalton, H.L. "AIDS in Black Face." Daedulus. Spring 1989.

286 Thomas, S.B. and Crouse Quinn, S. November 1991. op cit.

287 National Commission on AIDS. "America Living with AIDS: Transforming Anger, Fear, and Indifference into Action." Washington, D.C. September 1991.

288 Mays, V.M. and Cochran, S.D. 1988. op cit.

289 Airhihenbuwa, C.O. (in press) op cit.

290 Mays, V.M. and Cochran, S.D. 1988. op cit.

291 Rowell, R.M. "Native Americans, Stereotypes, and HIV/AIDS." SIECUS REPORT. Vol. 18. 1990.

292 Witcher, S. U.S. Department of Commerce, Bureau of the Census. Personal Communication. 1992.

293 Rowell, R.M. 1990. op cit.

294 Rowell, R.M. 1990. op cit.

295 Blum, R. 1992. op cit.

296 Blum, R. 1992. op cit.

297 Mays, V.M. and Cochran, S.D. 1988; Winett, R.A. 1986. op cit.

298 Intergovernmental Health Policy Project. "AIDS in Racial Minorities: A Challenge for State and Local Policymakers." George Washington University. Washington, D.C. 1990.

299 Peterson, J.L. "Issues in the Prevention of AIDS among Black and Hispanic Men." American Psychologist. Vol. 43. No. 11. 1988.

300 Office of Minority Health. 1990. op cit.

301 National Commission on AIDS. March 1991. op cit.

302 Fullilove, M.T., et al. "Shaping AIDS Education and Prevention Programs for African Americans Amidst Community Decline." Journal of Negro Education. Vol. 60. No. 1. 1991.

303 CDC. January 13, 1992. op cit.

304 CDC. Special Report on Evaluation. HIV/AIDS Prevention. February 1991.

305 Miller, H.G., et al. 1990. op cit.

306 CDC. February 1991. op cit.

307 Overby, K.J., et al. "Knowledge and Concerns about AIDS and Their Relationship to Behavior among Adolescents with Hemophilia." Pediatrics. Vol. 83. No. 2. 1989.

308 Goldsmith, M.F. "Medical News and Perspectives: Target: Sexually Transmitted Diseases." Journal of the American Medical Association. Vol. 264. 1990.

309 Mason, P.J., et al. "AIDS, Hemophilia, and Prevention Efforts Within a Comprehensive Care Program." American Psychologist. Vol. 43. No. 11. November 1988.

310 Mason, P.J., et al. 1988. op cit.

311 Overby, K.J., et al. 1989. op cit.

312 CDC. HIV/AIDS Prevention Newsletter. Vol. 2. No. 3. December 1991.

313 National Center for Education in Maternal and Child Health. Pediatric AIDS: Abstracts of Active Projects, FY1990 and FY1991. Washington, D.C. 1991.

314 Miller, H.G., et al. (eds.) 1990. op cit.

315 Miller, H.G., et al. (eds.) 1990. op cit.

316 U.S. Department of Health and Human Services. National Center on Child Abuse and Neglect (NCCAN). *Research Symposium on Child Sexual Abuse*. May 1988.

317 The National Committee for the Prevention of Child Abuse (NCPCA). The National Center on Child Abuse Prevention Research. *Current Trends in Child Abuse Reporting and Fatalities: The Results of the 1990 Annual Fifty State Survey*. April 1991.

318 Harrison, P.A., et al. "Sexual Abuse Correlates: Similarities Between Male and Female Adolescents in Chemical Dependency Treatment." *Journal of Adolescent Health*. Vol. 4. No. 3. July 1989.

319 Zierler, S., et al. "Adult Survivors of Childhood Sexual Abuse and Subsequent Risk of HIV Infection." *American Journal of Public Health*. Vol 81. No. 5. May 1991.

320 Burgess, A.W. and Hartman, C.R. "AIDS and the Sexually Abused Adolescent." *Troubled Adolescents and HIV Infection: Issues in Prevention and Treatment*. Child and Adolescent Service System Program (CASSP). October 1989.

321 Gutman, L.T., et al. "Human Immunodeficiency Virus Transmission by Child Sexual Abuse." *American Journal of Diseases of Children*. Vol. 145. February 1991.

322 Boyer, D. and Fine, D. "Sexual Abuse as a Factor in Adolescent Pregnancy and Child Maltreatment." *Family Planning Perspectives*. Vol. 24. No. 1. Jan./Feb. 1992; Finkelhor, D., et al. "Sexual Abuse and its Relationship to Later Sexual Satisfaction, Marital Status, Religion, and Attitudes." *Journal of Interpersonal Violence*. Vol. 4. No. 4. December 1989.

323 Miller, H.G., et al. (eds.) 1990. op cit.; Rotheram-Borus, M.J. June 1991. op cit.; Personal Communications with Shoshanna Rosenfeld and Deborah Lewis, 1990.

324 Zierler, S., et al. 1991. op cit.

325 Boyer, D. and Fine, D. 1992. op cit.

326 Riggs. S., et al. "Health Risk Behaviors and Attempted Suicide in Adolescents Who Report Prior Maltreatment." The Journal of Pediatrics. Vol. 116. 1990.

327 Finkelhor, D., et al. 1989. op cit.; De Young, M. The Sexual Victimization of Children. Jefferson, North Carolina: McFarland & Company, Inc. 1982; Cavaiola, A.A., and Schiff, M. "Behavioral Sequelae of Physical and/or Sexual Abuse in Adolescents." Child Abuse and Neglect. Vol. 12. 1988.

328 Harrison, P.A., et al. July 1989. op cit.

329 Singer, M.I., et al. "The Relationship Between Sexual Abuse and Substance Abuse Among Psychiatrically Hospitalized Adolescents." Child Abuse and Neglect. Vol. 13. 1989; Cavaiola, A.A. and Schiff, M. 1988. op cit.; Riggs S., et al. 1990. op cit.

330 Spatz-Widom, C. "Childhood Victimization and Adolescent Problem Behaviors." Paper presented at National Institute of Child Health and Human Development Conference. Adolescent Problems and Risk-Taking Behaviors. Berkeley Springs, West Virginia. April 1991.

331 Spatz-Widom, C. April 1991. op cit.

332 Spatz-Widom, C. April 1991. op cit.

CHAPTER IV

ADOLESCENTS FACE NUMEROUS BARRIERS TO RECEIVING HIV-RELATED CARE AND SERVICES†

The burgeoning HIV epidemic has dramatized the plight of many Americans who are uninsured or underinsured, and who lack access to adequate health care and other services. Adolescents confront numerous obstacles to receiving HIV-related care and services, including financial barriers, lack of adequately trained providers, a fragmented health-care delivery system, and unresolved legal and ethical considerations. As observed by Jean Garrison Athey, Chief of the Public Health Social Work Division within the Bureau of Maternal and Child Health:

> ...There are problems and limitations in the current array of health, mental health, and social services for adolescents. Attitudinal, political/administrative, financial, and legal barriers all negatively affect service delivery. As a result, the availability of services is uneven; services are frequently inappropriate and insensitive and thus unacceptable to many adolescents; and services are often fragmented, leading to difficulties in access both within and across systems. These service failures become especially apparent when an adolescent acquires HIV infection. Youth at highest risk for contracting HIV appear to be those who are least well-served by the traditional health, mental health, and social service systems.[1]

A recent report by a panel of the Department of Health and Human Services, chaired by the Surgeon General, described the wide range of services that children with HIV-infection or AIDS and their families may need, including: integrated medical care; mental health assessments and interventions; drug treatment; HIV-antibody testing and counseling; housing; legal services; primary prevention; education and behavior change; developmental services; special and school-based education; family-to-family support; nutrition assistance; foster care; adoption services; and group care.[2]

---

† Excerpted from CRS Report 102-1074

The range and availability of services required for adolescents infected with HIV or at risk of infection have essentially not been discussed in any systematic fashion.[3] However, many of the services identified by the PHS Panel as necessary for children are also likely to be required for adolescents with HIV infection and AIDS and their families.

While access to the full range of legal, housing, and other support services is critical to adolescents with HIV infection or AIDS, the remainder of this chapter will focus primarily on barriers to medical care, HIV-antibody testing and counseling, and education.

A. FINANCIAL BARRIERS TO HIV-RELATED HEALTH CARE

Cost of HIV-Related Treatment for Youth Unknown

Cost estimates for treating people with HIV disease and AIDS vary considerably. According to the Congressional Research Service, average health care expenditures between the time of AIDS diagnosis and death have ranged from $24,000 - $147,000.[4] In June 1986, the Public Health Service's "Coolfont" report projected that the annual cost of treatment for all individuals with AIDS or HIV infection in Fiscal Year 1991 would be $8-16 billion.[5]

More recently, a study by the Agency for Health Care Policy and Research (AHCPR), estimates that the cost of treating all people with HIV and AIDS will be $5.8 billion in 1991, reaching $10.4 billion in 1994.[6] AHCPR estimates that the average annual cost of treating a person with AIDS is $32,000, and for treating a person with HIV infection, but not AIDS, is $5,150. AHCPR also estimates that the average cost of treatment between AIDS diagnosis and death is more than $85,000.

Estimates of the cost of treating adolescents and young adults with HIV disease and AIDS are not available, but if we consider the number of teens currently infected with HIV and those at risk of infection, potential costs could prove overwhelming.

Adolescents with Private Health Insurance Still Face Barriers to HIV-Related Care

Adolescents' access to health care depends to a great extent on whether they have health insurance. In 1988, nearly 70% of U.S. adolescents ages 10-18 were covered at least partially by private health insurance.[7] Most adolescents who have private health insurance are covered as dependents under their parents' employer-based plans.[8] The benefits available to privately insured youth depend on the type of insurance and the terms of the insurance policy.

Comprehensive national data on benefit coverage are fairly limited, and to date there have been no surveys of private health insurance benefits that have focussed specifically on adolescent needs.[9] In general, according to OTA and the American Medical Association (AMA), adolescents with private health insurance are well covered for traditional medical services such as hospital care, physician services, and prescription medicines.[10] Compared with these services, private insurance is less likely to cover preventive and case management services for adolescents, and most private policies limit inpatient and outpatient mental health and substance abuse treatment services - two of the services that teens with HIV or at risk of infection are likely to need the most.[11]

As noted by OTA, "employer and insurer attitudes toward coverage of mental health and substance abuse treatment are in flux, especially with respect to adolescents."[12] Utilization of these services increased dramatically during the last decade, and many employers and private insurers are reconsidering how and whether to cover mental health and drug abuse treatment benefits for dependents.[13] OTA also found that according to a recent survey of corporate benefits decision makers, more than half predicted restricting or excluding dependent coverage for these services.[14] These findings are particularly disturbing because as found previously in this report, of the estimated 1.6 million adolescents who needed drug treatment in 1989, only 123,500 actually received it.

Cost of Treating People with HIV and AIDS Increasingly Born by Public Health Insurance; One in Three Poor Teens Not Eligible for Medicaid

People with AIDS and HIV infection face serious barriers to obtaining adequate health insurance coverage.[15] Since the mid-1980s, the responsibility for paying the cost of AIDS treatment has gradually shifted from private to public health insurance programs.[16] This change reflects a shift in the demographics of the HIV-infected population, which is increasingly poor and without health insurance.[17]

Early studies found that private health insurance covered 40% to 60% of total costs associated with HIV-related treatment, while Medicaid covered an additional 20% to 30% and Medicare paid 1% to 3%. In recent years, however, Medicaid has covered an increasing share of the HIV-related health care costs, particularly for expenditures related to inpatient care.[18]

An estimated 4.6 million U.S. adolescents ages 10 to 18 had Medicaid coverage at some time during FY 1988, the most recent year for which data are available.[19] The number of youth with HIV disease or AIDS who were served is uncertain and Medicaid expenditures for adolescents with AIDS are not available.[20] It is likely, however, that Medicaid is an important player in treating adolescents with HIV and AIDS.

Within broad Federal guidelines, each state determines not only the criteria for Medicaid eligibility, but also the services it will provide. Therefore, the benefits available to Medicaid-eligible adolescents with HIV or AIDS depend to a great extent on the state in which that individual resides.[21]

State Medicaid programs must cover a core of essential services including, but not limited to: inpatient and outpatient hospital services; physician services; early and periodic screening, diagnosis, and treatment (EPSDT); laboratory and x-ray procedures; and family planning services and supplies.[22] States may also opt to cover other services including case management, prescribed drugs, home health care, and hospice care. At least four states (AL, MD, PA, and WA) have added targeted case management to the services available to Medicaid-eligible persons with HIV or AIDS.[23]

In 1989, Congress significantly expanded adolescents' access to Medicaid-covered services by reforming the EPSDT program within Medicaid.[24] States are now mandated to periodically screen Medicaid-eligible adolescents under age 22 for any illnesses, abnormalities, or treatable conditions and refer them for definitive treatment.[25] In addition, states are now required to provide any federally reimbursable service that is "medically necessary" to diagnose or treat a problem identified in an EPSDT screening, regardless of whether that service is included in the state's Medicaid plan.[26]

States are permitted to set limits on the number of screenings that will be covered by their EPSDT programs. In 1989, only 22 states[(a)] offered five or more scheduled EPSDT screenings for youth ages 10 to 21, compared with four states (ID, OK, TX, and WY) which covered only one or two visits. Minnesota covered as many EPSDT visits as were "medically necessary."[27]

While the expansion of the EPSDT program may potentially assist HIV-infected, Medicaid-eligible adolescents to receive care, this potential will not be realized unless adolescents are actually screened.[28] In fact, since the law was enacted, states have made little progress in enrolling Medicaid-eligible children in the EPSDT program.[29]

States have the option to request waivers to provide a broader range of home and community-based services to individuals with HIV infection and AIDS than would normally be available under their Medicaid plan.[30] By February 1991,

---

(a) States that offered five or more EPSDT screening for ages 10-21 in 1989: AL; DE; FL; GA; HI; IL; IN; ME; MD; MA; MI; NE; NY; ND; OH; OR; PA; RI; VT; WA; WV: and WI.

AIDS-specific waivers had been approved for 15 states[(b)] and 24 states had opted to cover hospice benefits for Medicaid-eligible persons with terminal illness.[31] The effectiveness of these programs in meeting the needs of HIV-infected adolescents depends on the specific provisions of each state's program.[32]

While the Medicaid program has the potential to assist many HIV-infected adolescents, it is important to note that one in three poor adolescents ages 10-18 (1.76 million) was neither eligible for Medicaid nor covered by private health insurance in 1988.[33]

Due to changes in Federal law enacted in 1990, Medicaid eligibility has been expanded to gradually phase in, one year at a time, coverage to children ages seven through 18 who are in families with incomes below the Federal poverty level.[34] This expansion will certainly assist numerous children. However, it is unlikely to help adolescents for a number of years. All poor adolescents under age 19 will not become eligible for Medicaid until October 2001.[35]

<u>**Millions of Adolescents Lack Private Health Insurance and Are Not Eligible for Medicaid**</u>

Between 1979 and 1986, the percentage of adolescents ages 10-18 without health insurance increased by 25%.[36] (Due to modifications in the questionnaire, survey data from 1979 to 1986 cannot be compared with more recent data.[37]) The percent of uninsured adolescents continued to increase between 1987 and 1988 by an estimated 5%, paralleling an overall increase in the nonelderly population without health insurance.[38]

By 1988, an estimated one in seven adolescents ages 10-18 (4.6 million or 15% of the U.S. population ages 10-18) lacked private health insurance and remained ineligible for Medicaid because of family income or minor status.[39] Young adults under

---

(b) The 15 states included CA, CO, DE, FL, HI, IL, IA, MO NJ, NM, OH, PA, SC, VA, and WA. Illinois and North Carolina also include persons with AIDS under similar waivers for broader populations.

age 25, who more likely than young adolescents to be infected with HIV, are even less likely to be privately insured or eligible for public assistance. An estimated 27.4% of young adults ages 18-24 lacked health insurance in 1989.[40]

Uninsured adolescents tend to be in poorer health, wait longer periods of time between physician visits, and are more likely to be hospitalized, due in part to delays in seeking medical care.[41] Poor adolescents, minority youth, and those that have runaway or are homeless or incarcerated are at especially high risk of being uninsured.[42] As found previously, many of these youth are also more likely to have AIDS, to be infected with HIV, and are at increased risk of infection.

B. LACK OF ADEQUATELY TRAINED HEALTH CARE PROVIDERS AND POOR DISTRIBUTION OF COMMUNITY AND PUBLIC HEALTH PROGRAMS THREATEN QUALITY OF CARE AVAILABLE TO HIV-INFECTED YOUTH

Adolescents are less likely to utilize private office-based primary care physicians than any other age group.[43] A number of nonfinancial and nonlegal reasons account for low utilization of services by primary care physicians, and to some extent other health care providers. According to OTA, these include: the lack of availability and willingness of physicians to treat adolescents; inconsistencies between adolescents' perceived needs and the care provided by physicians; adolescents' concerns about confidentiality; and physicians' and other health care providers' lack of competence to identify and treat the health problems of adolescents.[44]

The majority of U.S. adolescents who obtain medical care receive it from providers who have not received special training in adolescent health.[45] There are no definitive data on the number of physicians who specialize in adolescent medicine. However, available data indicate that the number of physicians who dedicate their practices to adolescent medicine is quite small.[46] The American Medical Association (AMA) estimates that there is only one adolescent medicine specialist for every 20,500 adolescents, and one child and adolescent psychiatrist for every 5,000 adolescents. Only 1,261 of the nearly 800,000 members of the American Medical Association selected adolescent medicine as a primary or secondary specialty.[47]

The Society for Adolescent Medicine (SAM) claimed just over 1,034 members in 1989, while in 1988, the American Academy of Pediatrics' Section on Adolescent Health included only 547 members, of whom the vast majority (an estimated 500) were <u>also</u> members of the Society for Adolescent Medicine.[48]

The lack of adequately trained adolescent health care providers is even more pronounced for adolescents with HIV infection. According to Karen Hein, who directs one of the few comprehensive adolescent AIDS treatment programs in the United States, there is an urgent need for:

> ...developing HIV specific programs for teenagers by training or revamping adolescent providers, [including] adolescent medicine specialists, family practitioners, and pediatricians, for example, to be able to provide HIV expertise, <u>and</u> [for] revamping HIV/AIDS specialists, [including] infectious diseases specialists, hematologists, and immunologists, for example, to be knowledgeable about the adolescent.[49]

Federally funded community and migrant health centers, health care for the homeless clinics, and family planning clinics play a critical role in delivering HIV-related information and health care services to poor and medically underserved adolescents.

Approximately 550 community and migrant health centers (CHCs and MHCs) provide direct comprehensive primary care services to approximately 6.3 million medically underserved persons. An estimated 44% of the persons treated by CHCs and MHCs are children under age 18. Approximately 2% to 4% of the population seen by these centers is infected with HIV.[50] Clinics receiving Health Care for the Homeless funds (Section 340 of the Public Health Service Act) also serve medically underserved adolescents. In FY 1989, an estimated 17,600 adolescents ages 15-19 received services from these clinics.[51]

Similarly, federally funded (Title X) family planning clinics are located in all 50 states and in two-thirds of counties.[52] The number of adolescents served by federally funded clinics is uncertain. The most recent available data indicated that approximately one-third of the 4.1 million women who were served in 1981 were teens.[53] Federally funded family planning clinics provide a variety of services including family planning, contraceptive services, and STD and HIV screening. In 1989 and 1990, 15 percent of the HIV tests that were conducted by publicly funded clinics were provided at family planning clinics.[54]

Despite their immense potential to reach millions of adolescents who are not served by private physicians, funding for CHCs, MHC, and Title X has decreased during the past decade. Between 1980 and 1991, funding for CHCs and MHCs declined by 2.4% and funding for Title X decreased by 61%, adjusted for inflation.[55]

C. HIV INFECTION AMONG ADOLESCENTS RAISES COMPLEX LEGAL AND ETHICAL ISSUES[(c)]

The growing HIV epidemic has raised complex legal and ethical issues for those living with the virus and its related illnesses, as well as for society at-large. These issues include: HIV-antibody testing and screening; consent and access to medical treatment; privacy rights; protection against discrimination; duty to warn; types and content of educational interventions; and liability. Gostin's 1990 review of 469 cases completed or pending before Federal, state or local courts and commissions notes:

> No other infectious disease in recent history compares with human immunodeficiency virus (HIV) infection in the ways it has affected our relationships with each other and with our social institutions. Sharp differences in perception of

---

(c) This section updates information and case law provided in the Select Committee on Children, Youth, and Families' 1987 report, A Generation in Jeopardy: Children and AIDS. The content was developed with the assistance of the Congressional Research Service's American Law Division, in conformance with a request from the Select Committee, but does not necessarily represent the opinion of CRS.

public health, ethics, and civil liberties have created the largest body of legal cases attributable to a single disease in the history of American jurisprudence.[56]

Since much of the attention to the AIDS crisis has focused on adults, the majority of legal cases have been brought on behalf of adult claimants. Nevertheless, questions have been raised specifically on behalf of youth and many cases and resulting judgments concerning adults have application to adolescents.[57]

Legal and ethical concerns often become more complicated when considering children and youth affected by the epidemic. A hodgepodge of laws and policies at the Federal, state and local levels affects young people, and more gaps exist than are filled.[58] The circumstances of adolescents pose especially difficult challenges. Adolescents generally receive less attention and fewer resources devoted to their particular needs.

Adolescents are undergoing dramatic and rapid physical and psychological changes as they develop their own identities and independence. Just as the design of appropriate and effective prevention and treatment services needs to take into account adolescent development, legal and ethical considerations "cannot simply rely on the perspectives which are appropriate either for adults or for young children."[59]

When the Committee first investigated HIV and adolescents in 1987, Hein posed several ethical and legal questions that remain relevant today:

> Do adolescents have the right as minor[s] to participate in screening if it were available?...If they are screened, do they have the right not to be told the results? Should they have access to anonymous testing?...Should parents be involved, again, in the decision to be tested? What about if, at result time, the results are positive, should parents be notified? If so, this would be quite different from other STDs....How can we inform immature minors about the issues involved in testing and in being positive? What about their partners who, themselves, are minors? What about case contacting?[60]

English and others continue to raise additional questions, many of which remain unanswered:

> Can an adolescent independently consent to an HIV antibody test, without parental permission? What is the scope of the confidentiality protection for an institutionalized adolescent known to be infected with the virus? Who, if anyone, is liable if an adolescent suffering from AIDS engages in sexual activity, or shares needles with a drug using companion, while in a group placement under public agency supervision? Can educational or social services programs legally refuse to serve infected youth?[61]
>
> Who, if anyone, is liable if disclosure of an adolescent's antibody status results in discrimination or other harm to the adolescent?[62]

This section examines legal and ethical issues in three principal areas: (1) issues of HIV testing and medical treatment that arise and are of particular concern because of the age and legal status of the adolescent; (2) privacy issues; and (3) issues concerning discrimination.

HIV-Antibody Testing and Medical Treatment Should Be Inextricably Linked

Early detection of HIV has become increasingly important as early prophylactic treatment has the potential to delay onset of symptoms of HIV disease and/or prolong the lives of those individuals who have become infected. As noted by English, "voluntary HIV testing is increasingly considered a gateway to treatment and something to be encouraged for individuals who are at risk of infection."[63]

Problems associated with adolescents' access to health care in general, along with the scarcity of HIV specific services for teens, make the necessary linkage between access to care and HIV-antibody testing difficult to achieve for adolescents, particularly those at highest risk of infection.[64] As noted by Rotheram-Borus, "No resources are associated with the increased demand for testing, so that many problems emerge."[65]

Authority for Decision-Making

Questions arise about who has decision-making authority concerning the testing and treatment of adolescents who are considered minor children (under age 18 in most states). Some adolescents may not seek care unless they can obtain it independently.[66] Under current laws in all 50 states, the District of Columbia, and Puerto Rico, minors have authority to consent to certain kinds of medical treatment without parental consent, although the laws vary widely.[67]

As noted by English:

> Although the law generally requires parental consent when health care is provided to minor children, there are numerous exceptions -- based on the minor's status or the specific services sought.[68]

Further, North found:

> The statutory exceptions to the need for parental consent vary substantially from state to state, but generally fall within two categories: (1) those that authorize a minor to consent to specific types of care, such as treatment of venereal disease, drug abuse, pregnancy, or injury resulting from an alleged rape or sex offense, or even HIV testing; and (2) those that authorize certain minors to consent to all care based upon the minor's competence or maturity.[69]

As shown in Table 1 below, according to a recent review by English, at least 11 states have statutes which explicitly give minors authority to consent to HIV testing.[70] Only three of these states also explicitly authorize minors to consent for treatment for AIDS or HIV infection. Moreover, at least 12 states classify HIV infection or AIDS as an STD or venereal disease which would allow minors to consent to HIV diagnosis or treatment. Further, in at least nine states, minors are authorized to consent to testing and treatment for HIV or AIDS as a reportable, contagious, infectious, or communicable disease.[71]

Table 1: States with Specific Statutes Authorizing Minors to Consent for HIV-Antibody Testing and HIV-Related Treatment[d]

States with Specific Statute Authorizing Minors To Consent for HIV Testing		States with Specific Statute Authorizing Minors To Consent To Treatment for AIDS or HIV	States with Specific Authorizing Minors To Consent To Testing and Treatment To Testing and STD		States with Specific Statutory Authority for Minors To Consent To Testing And Treatment for HIV or AIDS as Reportable, Contagious Infectious, or Communicable Disease	
Arizona	Montana	Colorado	Alabama	Nevada	Alabama	Oklahoma
California	New Mexico	Iowa	Florida	South Carolina	California	Pennsylvania
Colorado	New York	Michigan	Illinois	Tennessee	Idaho	Texas
Delaware	Ohio		Kentucky	Vermont	Montana	Virginia
Iowa	Wisconsin		Mississippi	Washington	North Carolina	
Michigan			Montana	Wyoming		

(d) COMPILED FROM: English, Abigail. "Adolescents and HIV: Legal and Ethical Issues." National Center for Youth Law. San Francisco, California. Prepared for the Public Health Service Panel on Women, Adolescents, and Children with HIV Infection and AIDS and the Working Group on Legal and Ethical Issues Related to HIV of the Public Health Service Task Force. 1992. Statute citations appended in Table 2.

NOTE: Statutes reported by September 1991. Even in States without the explicit statutory authority summarized in this Table, some minors may be able to consent to HIV testing or treatment on the basis that they are runaways, homeless youth, mature minors, emancipated minors, high school graduates, pregnant minors, or minor parents. (English, 1992; North, 1990; Gittler, 1990.)

As noted in Table 1, many states also authorize some minors to consent to HIV-antibody testing and HIV-related treatment on the basis that they are runaways, homeless youth, mature minors, emancipated minors, high school graduates, pregnant minors, or minor parents.[72]

In order to improve access to treatment, efforts have been made to secure increased participation of adolescents in clinical trials and other research protocols, raising additional questions about consent authority.[73] Authority to consent to HIV testing and/or treatment does not convey independent authority for a minor to participate in research. As Melton has pointed out:

> Parents must give permission (distinguished from consent) before their children may participate in research, but in most instances minors retain power of assent (essentially, a veto power).[74]

English further describes that:

> ...if, under state law, minors may consent to HIV testing and/or treatment or if the adolescent research subjects are capable of giving informed consent -- and may therefore be considered "mature minors" -- and the research does not entail more than minimal risk, the requirement of parental permission may be waived....The regulations explicitly require that when parental permission is waived an alternative mechanism for protecting the children (or adolescents) must be substituted. The specific mechanism must be designed based on the particular risks involved in the research as well as the maturity and other characteristics of the adolescents who are the research subjects. Moreover, if the subjects of research are wards of the state or any agency or institution, and the research involves greater than minimal risk and no prospect of direct benefit, an advocate (in addition to anyone acting as guardian or *in loco parentis*) must be appointed to protect the best interests of each child or adolescent who is a research subject.[75]

HIV-antibody testing in general, and in particular for minor adolescents, remains controversial because of very limited pre- and post-test counseling services and privacy concerns, including potential breaches in confidentiality that can lead to stigmatization and discrimination against HIV-infected persons.[76] According to Hein, mandatory testing remains widely opposed by health care and service professionals "on the basis of invasion of privacy or of the civil rights of the individuals involved, lack of evidence that mandatory testing helps curtail the epidemic, and cost considerations."[77]

In her 1987 testimony, Shafer noted:

> Regarding testing, especially with adolescents, I have a big concern....If you require and mandate testing, that may backfire in that the groups that you want to reach with the counseling...to essentially change behaviors...won't enter the system and get that really in-depth counseling that's required.[78]

Similarly, Hein observes:

> Additional concerns apply to youths involved in the mandatory testing policies in the Job Corps or in the Military. Mandatory testing might make sense if it allowed youths to receive care earlier or in a more efficient or humane way, but mandatory HIV testing policies that are used to exclude HIV-positive applicants (as in the case of the military) or fail to provide adequate services (as charged in the law suit against the Job Corps) only exacerbate already inadequate services for disadvantaged youths.[79]

Mark presented another point of view in his 1987 testimony before the Committee. Mark suggested that repeated HIV testing is needed for epidemiologic purposes to see how far, and into which groups of the population, the HIV epidemic is spreading.[80] Others have pointed out to the Committee that seroprevalence studies for purposes of epidemiology can be done through unlinked anonymous testing. They note that if such a strategy is used, the adolescents who participate in unlinked seroprevalence studies should be offered with voluntary confidential testing with age-appropriate pre- and posttest counseling.[81]

In March 1988, the first conference ever to focus on AIDS and HIV among adolescents was held in New York City. At that meeting, experts from the Society for Adolescent Medicine and five Federal agencies developed a set a general principles and recommendations regarding the HIV-antibody testing and epidemiology which remain helpful today.[82] Following is the set of "General Principles" developed at that meeting:

1. Any HIV testing of adolescents should occur based only on expected benefits to adolescents.

2. There should be no mandatory HIV testing of population groups or individual adolescents as a prerequisite for admission to programs, services, or placements.

3. There should be no "routine" HIV testing, and especially no involuntary routine HIV testing, of adolescents.

4. When HIV testing is indicated, based on clinical criteria or an appropriate request of an adolescent, it should be conducted in settings where pre- and posttest counseling that is sensitive, age appropriate, and culturally appropriate is available.

5. In many situations, and especially in the case of a positive test result, the identification and participation of a supportive adult in the testing procedure and in follow-up care should be strongly encouraged.

6. Adolescents who are capable of giving an informed consent should be able to consent to an HIV test when pre- and posttest counseling and other appropriate safeguards are in place.

7. Maintaining confidentiality of HIV testing information concerning adolescents in conformity with both legal and the highest ethical standards is essential.

8. Special sensitivity is required with respect to the risk of coercion and loss of confidentiality in specialized settings, such as detention facilities, and special safeguards should be employed to ensure that this does not occur.

9. In order to define the extent of HIV infection among adolescents there is a need for targeted seroprevalence studies, from which the information should be used to

develop programs of prevention and services to direct future research.

10. Testing guidelines should be reviewed, and modified if necessary, on an ongoing basis dependent on the outcome of research studies of the impact of HIV testing on adolescents and other pertinent issues.[83]

Building on these guidelines and the recommendations that also were developed at that meeting, the Massachusetts Department of Public Health produced model guidelines for adolescent HIV-antibody counseling and testing that detail the risks and benefits of HIV-antibody testing. These guidelines, approved by the Governor, also provide protocols for pre- and posttest counseling sessions.[84]

Privacy

One of the main issues raised by HIV-antibody testing is the question of the right of privacy for the person tested. This issue involves questions regarding Federal and state constitutional rights, statutory provisions and common law principles. Legally, the degree of confidentiality protection and the scope of permissible disclosure may turn on numerous factors, including whether testing is voluntary or mandatory, whether there is consent to disclose results, the purpose of disclosure, and the application of specific statutory provisions. The issue has sometimes been seen in terms of balancing the individual's right to privacy against the need for society to know.

The public health community has generally agreed on the need for some type of confidentiality. For example, with regard to school-aged children, the CDC and the American Academy of Pediatrics (AAP) recommend that school and health officials respect the right to privacy of any student infected with the AIDS virus.[85]

In their 1985 Recommendations and Guidelines, CDC states:

> Parents of infected children should be aware of the potential for social isolation should the condition of the child become known to others in the care or educational setting. School,

> day-care and social service personnel and others involved in educating and care for these children should be sensitive to the need for confidentiality and the right to privacy in these cases.[86]

According to the AAP:

> The number of personnel aware of the child's condition should be kept to the minimum needed to assure proper care of the child and to detect situations in which the potential for transmission may increase.[87]

The rapidly evolving nature of the AIDS epidemic among adolescents suggests the importance of advice given by English, urging "very careful development and evaluation of any recommendations specific to children and youth."[88]

Nondiscrimination and Access to Schools

Prevention of discrimination against HIV-infected adults has been the subject of considerable discussion which contributed to the enactment of the Americans with Disabilities Act (ADA) on July 26, 1990.[(e)] The ADA provides broad-based nondiscrimination protection for individuals with disabilities in employment, public services, public accommodations and services operated by private entities, transportation, and telecommunications.

Although the statutory language of the ADA does not specifically include HIV-infected persons, the Act was clearly intended to cover such individuals. The definition of individuals with disabilities is a functional one: the term disability is defined as meaning with respect to an individual "(A) a physical or mental impairment that substantially limits one or more of the major life activities of such individual; (B) a record of such an impairment; or (C) being regarded as having such an impairment." The Senate Report on the ADA discussed the meaning of the definition and stated "... a person infected with the Human Immunodeficiency Virus is covered under the first prong of the definition of the term 'disability'."[(f)]

(e) P.L. 101-336, 42 U.S.C. §§ 12101 *et seq.*

Similarly, the ADA also was intended to cover youth as well as children and adults. The definition as cited above does not contain any age related requirement and clearly some of the public services and places of public accommodation would be used by youth. The Senate Report confirms this view in its discussion of school bus requirements under title II of the Act when it states that "equal nonsegregated opportunities are provided to all children."[g]

Two other Federal statutes could provide significant protection for HIV-infected youth: section 504 of the Rehabilitation Act of 1973;[h] and the Individuals with Disabilities Education Act (IDEA).[i] Although section 504, like the ADA, could be a source for rights of youth in areas such as employment, transportation, and access to child welfare services and residential placements, the primary import of all of these statutes for youth so far has been with respect to access to education. Before analyzing this particular legal issue, it is helpful to note that CDC has published guidelines concerning access to education.

CDC, along with many state education and health departments, has recommended that most youth infected with

---

(f) U.S. Senate Report 101-116, 101st Congress, First Session. 1989

(g) Id.

(h) 29 U.S.C. § 794. Section 504 prohibits discrimination against otherwise qualified handicapped individuals solely by reason of their handicap in any program or activity that receives federal financial assistance or in the executive agencies or the United States Postal Service. The ADA was modeled on section 504 and expanded its nondiscrimination requirements into the private sector; that is, those entities not covered under section 504 because they do not receive federal financial assistance.

(i) 20 U.S.C. §§ 1400 et seq. IDEA, formerly titled the Education for All Handicapped Children Act, authorizes a number of grant programs relating to the education of children with disabilities and requires that states receiving grants provide children with disabilities a free appropriate public education.

HIV be allowed to attend school. In its recommendations on education and foster care of HIV-infected children, CDC explains that none of the identified cases of HIV infection in the U.S. are known to have been transmitted in school or foster care settings or through casual person-to-person contact.[89]

Specifically, youth with HIV infection do not transmit the infection by sharing eating or drinking utensils, coughs or sneezes, or casual kissing on the cheeks or mouth. In addition, although HIV-infected youth may themselves face greater risk of infection in a group setting because of their immune system deficiencies, CDC has indicated that:

> For most infected school-aged children, the benefits of an unrestricted setting would outweigh the risks of their acquiring potential harmful infections in the setting and the apparent nonexistent risk of transmission. These youth should be allowed to attend school and after-school day-care and to be placed in a foster home in an unrestricted setting.[90]

The National Association of State Boards of Education reported that as of September 1987 a majority of states (39) had policies or a position statement on admitting students with AIDS to school.[91]

Guidelines issued by CDC note that decisions regarding the kind of educational and care setting for the child infected with the AIDS virus "should be based on the behavior, neurologic development, and physical condition of the child and the expected type of interaction with others in that setting," and that each case should be evaluated individually by a team that includes the child's physician, public health officials, the child's parent or guardian and personnel from the care facility or school.[92]

The ADA, section 504, and IDEA could be used as possible statutory bases for a right to education for HIV-infected youth. Both section 504 and the ADA prohibit discrimination against individuals with disabilities and it would appear to be fairly settled law that these statutes include HIV-infected individuals within their definitions of individuals with disabilities.[j] It is also fairly settled in case law that an automatic exclusion from school of HIV-infected children would violate section 504.[k]

In an analogous case involving a teacher with the contagious disease of tuberculosis, the Supreme Court held that the teacher may be a handicapped person under section 504, and that the fact of the possibility of contagion did not limit the coverage of the section. The Court further found that the issue of whether such contagious individuals are protected by section 504 is determined by whether such an individual is "otherwise qualified." In determining whether an individual is otherwise qualified, the Court found that an individualized inquiry must be made concerning the nature of the risk, the duration of the risk, the severity of the risk, and the probability that the disease will be transmitted. A court must then evaluate whether reasonable accommodation is possible. This same approach has been adopted in lower court cases involving HIV-infected children.[l]

IDEA could also be used as a basis for requiring the education of an HIV-infected adolescent. This Act provides federal funds to the states and conditions the receipt of these funds on the provision of a "free appropriate public education." It would appear that the Act would cover some HIV-infected children. Madeleine Will, former Assistant Secretary for Special Education and Rehabilitative Services, indicated that:

> [C]hildren with AIDS would be eligible for coverage under EHA-B if they are evaluated as having one of the handicapping conditions listed in the statute, and in need of

---

(j) School Board of Nassau County v. Arline, 480 U.S. 273 (1987); Thomas v. Atascadero Unified School District, 662 F.Supp. 376 (C.D. Calif. 1987); U.S. Department of Justice, "Application of Section 504 of the Rehabilitation Act to HIV-Infected Individuals," (September 27, 1988).

(k) Doe v. Dolton Elementary School District No. 148, 694 F.Supp. 440 (N.D. Ill. 1988); Thomas V. Atascadero Unified School District, 662 F.Supp. 376 (C.D. Calif. 1987).

(l) Doe v. Dolton Elementary School District. No. 148, 694 F.Supp. 440 (N.D. Ill. 1988).

special education and related services. Children with AIDS could be eligible for special education programs under the category of 'other health impaired'.[m]

(m) 221 EHLR 343 (1984).

Table 2:	State Laws Authorizing Minors to Consent for HIV-Antibody Testing and HIV-Related Treatment[(n)]
Alabama	Rules of State Bd. of Health, Division of Disease Control § 420-4-1-03 (1987) [HIV classified as STD]; Ala. Code § 22-11A-19 (Supp. 1989) [minors may consent to STD care]); Ala. Code § 22-11A-14 (1984) [HIV is reportable disease]; Ala. Code § 22-8-6 (1984) [minors of any age may consent to diagnosis and treatment of reportable diseases].
Arizona	Ariz. Rev. Stat. Ann. §§ 36-661(2) and 36-663 (Supp. 1990) [written informed consent required for and HIV test; capacity to consent determined without regard to age].
California	Cal. Health and Safety Code §§ 199.22 and 199.27(a)(West 1990) [written consent of competent subject of HIV antibody test required; minors under age 12 deemed incompetent to consent to test]; 17 Cal. Code Reg. 17, § 2500 (4-1-90) [AIDS is reportable communicable disease]; Cal. Civ. Code § 34.7 (West 1982) [minors age 12 or older may consent to diagnosis and treatment of reportable infectious, contagious, or communicable diseases].
Colorado	Colo. Rev. Stat. Ann. § 25-4-1405(6) (1990) [minor may be examined and treated for HIV infection without consent of a parent]; Colo. Rev. Stat. Ann. § 25-4-1405(6) (1990).
Delaware	Del. Code Ann. tit. 16, § 1202(f) (Supp. 1988) [minors age 12 and older may give informed consent for HIV testing and counseling].

[(n)] COMPILED FROM: English, Abigail. "Adolescents and HIV: Legal and Ethical Issues." National Center for Youth Law. San Francisco, California. Prepared for the Public Health Service Panel on Women, Adolescents, and Children with HIV Infection and AIDS and the Working Group on Legal and Ethical Issues Related to HIV of the Public Health Service Task Force. 1992.

NOTE: Statutes reported by September 1991. Even in states without the explicit statutory authority summarized in this Table, some minors may be able to consent to HIV testing or treatment on the basis that they are runaways, homeless youth, mature minors, emancipated minors, high school graduates, pregnant minors, or minor parents. (English, 1992; North 1990; Gittler 1990.)

Florida	Fla. Stat. Ann. § 384.23 (West Supp. 1991) [Department of Health shall consider HIV in designating STDs]; Fla. Stat. Ann. § 384.30 [minors may consent to confidential treatment for STDs].
Idaho	Idaho Code § 39-601 (1990) [AIDS, ARC and HIV classified as contagious, infectious and communicable]; Idaho Code § 39-3801 (Supp. 1988) [minors age 14 or older may consent to diagnosis and treatment of reportable infectious, contagious, or communicable diseases].
Iowa	Iowa Code Ann. § 144.22 (West Supp. 1991) [minor may apply and give consent for screening or treatment for AIDS]; Iowa Code Ann. § 144.22 (West Supp. 1991).
Illinois	Ill. Ann. Stat. ch. 111 1/2, para. 7403(3) (Smith-Hurd Supp. 1991) [HIV is classified as STD]; Ill. Ann. Stat. ch. 111, paras. 4504 and 4505 (Smith Hurd Supp. 1988) [minors age 12 or older may consent to VD diagnosis and treatment].
Kentucky	Ky. Rev. Stat. Ann. § 214.410 (Baldwin 1991) [STD defined to include AIDS and HIV]; Ky. Rev. Stat. Ann. § 214.185 (Baldwin 1982) [minors may consent to diagnosis and treatment of VD].
Michigan	Mich. Comp. Laws Ann. § 333.5127 (West Supp. 1991) [minor may consent to medical or surgical care, treatment or services for HIV]; Mich. Comp. Laws Ann. § 333.5127 (West Supp. 1991).
Mississippi	Miss. State Dept. Health 1990 List of Reportable Diseases [HIV classified as STD]; Miss. Code Ann. § 41-41-13 (1981) [minors may obtain treatment for VD without parental consent].
Montana	Mont. Code Ann. § 50-16-1007 (1989) [minors may consent for HIV related test]; Mont. Code Ann. § 50-18-101 (1989) [AIDS is defined as STD]; Mont. Admin. R. 16.28.204 (1987) [HIV is reportable]; Mont. Code Ann. § 41-1-402 (1989) [minors may consent to care for reportable STDs].

Nevada	P. Albert, R. Eisenberg, D.A. Hansell, J.K. Marcus (Eds.). (1991). <u>AIDS practice manual: A legal and educational guide</u> (3rd ed.) (App. A). San Francisco, CA: National Lawyers Guild AIDS Network. [HIV is classified as STD]; Nev. Rev. Stat. Ann. § 129.060 (Michie 1986) [minors may consent to examination and treatment for VD].
New Mexico	N.M. Stat. Ann. § 24-2B-3 (Supp. 1990) [minor has capacity to give informed consent for HIV test].
New York	N.Y. Pub. Health Law § 2780(5) and 2781(1) (McKinney Supp. 1991) [written informed consent required for an HIV related test; capacity to consent is determined without regard to age].
North Carolina	N.C. Gen. Stat. § 130A-135 (1989) [HIV is a reportable communicable condition]; N.C. Gen. Stat. § 90-21.5 (1985) [minors may consent to medical services to prevent, diagnose and treat reportable diseases].
Ohio	Ohio Rev. Code Ann. § 3701.242(B) (Page Supp. 1990) [minor may give consent for an HIV test].
Oklahoma	Oklahoma State Board of Health, Regulations for Reporting Cases of Disease, §§ 100 <u>et seq</u>. [HIV is reportable communicable disease]; Okla. Stat. Ann. tit. 63, § 2602 (1984) [minors may consent to treatment of reportable communicable diseases].
Pennsylvania	Pa. Stat. Ann. tit. 35, § 7607(9) (Purdon Supp. 1991) [HIV reporting to state permitted]; Pa. Stat. Ann. tit. 35, § 10103 (Purdon 1977) [minors may consent to treatment of reportable diseases].
South Carolina	S.C. Dept. Health 1990 List of Reportable Diseases and S.C. Code Ann. § 44-29-10, -70 (Law Co-op. Supp. 1989) [HIV is reportable STD]; S.C. Code Ann. § 20-7-280 (Law Co-op. 1985) [minors 16 or older may consent to any health services except operations]; S.C. Code Ann. § 20-7-290 (Law Co-op 1985) [minors of any age may receive without parental consent health services deemed by the provider necessary to maintain the well-being of the child].

Tennessee	AIDS practice manual (App. A) [HIV classified as STD]; Tenn. Code Ann. § 68-10-104 (1987) [minors may be examined, diagnosed and treated for VD without parental consent].
Texas	Tex. Health & Safety Code Ann. § 81.041(e) (Vernon 1991) [HIV and AIDS are reportable diseases]; Tex. Fam. Code Ann. § 35.03 (Vernon 1986) [minors may consent to treatment of reportable, infectious, contagious, or communicable diseases].
Vermont	Vt. Stat. Ann. tit. 18, § 1091 (1968) and AIDS practice manual (App. A) [HIV classified as HIV]; Vt. Stat. Ann. tit. 18, § 4226 (1982) [minors age 12 and older may consent to VD treatment].
Virginia	Va. Code Ann. § 32.1-116.3 (Supp. 1990) [HIV is defined as communicable disease for certain purposes]; Va. Code Ann. § 54.1-2969(D)(1) (1988) [minors may consent to diagnosis and treatment of any reportable infectious or contagious disease].
Washington	Wash. Rev. Code Ann. § 70.24.017 (Supp. 1991) [STD defined to include HIV and AIDS]; Wash. Rev. Code Ann. § 70.24.110 [minors age 14 and older may consent to diagnosis and treatment of STDs].
Wyoming	Wyo. Stat. § 35-4-130(b) (Supp. 1990) [AIDS defined as reportable STD]; Wyo. Stat. § 35-4-131 (1988) [minors may consent to examination and treatment for VD]. (Although the classification of HIV--as STD or VD--does not exactly match the designation of conditions--STD or VD--for which minors are authorized to consent to treatment in each of these states, it is likely that a court would broadly construe the minor consent statute to facilitate access to HIV-related care.)
Wisconsin	Wis. Stat. Ann. § 146.025(2)(a)(4) (West Supp. 1990) [consent of a competent minor age 14 or older is required for an HIV test].

Endnotes

1 Garrison, J. "Services and Treatment Issues: Recommendations of the Work Group." Journal of Adolescent Health Care. Vol. 10. No. 3. Supplement: "AIDS and Adolescents - Exploring the Challenge." 1989.

2 U.S. Department of Health and Human Services (DHHS). Panel on Women, Adolescents, and Children with HIV Infection and AIDS. "A Guide: Family-Centered Comprehensive Care for Children with HIV Infection." August 1991.

3 D'Angelo, L.J. and Sondheimer, D.L. "Adolescents and HIV Infection: Struggling Not to Be Forgotten." Pediatric AIDS. October 1990.

4 Merlis, M. Congressional Research Service (CRS). "Acquired Immune Deficiency Syndrome (AIDS): Health Care Financing and Services." Education and Public Welfare Division. December 31, 1990. Archived Issue Brief IB87219.

5 Institute of Medicine (IOM), National Academy of Sciences. "P.H.S. Plan for Prevention and Control of AIDS and the AIDS Virus." Confronting AIDS: Directions for Public Health, Health Care, and Research. Washington, D.C.: National Academy Press. 1986.

6 Hellinger, Fred J. "Forecasting the Medical Care Costs of the HIV Epidemic: 1991-1994." Agency for Health Care Policy and Research, Department of Health and Human Services. Inquiry. Vol. 28. No. 3. Fall 1991.

7 U.S. Congress. Office of Technology Assessment (OTA). Adolescent Health - Vol. III: Crosscutting Issues in the Delivery of Health and Related Services. Washington, D.C.: U.S. Government Printing Office. June 1991.

8 American Medical Association (AMA). AMA Profiles of Adolescent Health; Volume 2- Profiles of Adolescent Health Care; Use, Costs, and Problems of Access. 1991.

9 OTA. June 1991. op cit.

10 OTA. June 1991. op cit.; AMA. 1991. op cit.

11 AMA. 1991. op cit.

12 OTA. June 1991. op cit.

13 OTA. June 1991. op cit.

14 OTA. June 1991. op cit.

15 IOM. Report of a Study: The AIDS Research Program of the National Institutes of Health. Washington, D.C.: National Academy Press. March 1991; Merlis, M. (CRS). 1990. op cit.; National Commission on AIDS. America Living with AIDS - Transforming Anger, Fear, and Indifference into Action. Washington, D.C.: U.S. Government Printing Office. 1991.

16 Merlis, M. (CRS). 1990. op cit.; National Commission on AIDS. 1991. op cit.

17 IOM. March 1991. op cit.

18 Merlis, M. (CRS). 1990. op cit.

19 OTA. June 1991. op cit.

20 Merlis, M. (CRS). Education and Public Welfare Division. Personal communication. August 1991.

21 OTA. June 1991. op cit.

22 OTA. June 1991. op cit.

23 DHHS. August 1991. op cit.

24 Public Law 101-239, The Omnibus Budget Reconciliation Act of 1989. Sec. 6403.

25 Public Law 101-239. op cit.; OTA. June 1991. op cit.

26 Public Law 101-239. op cit.; English, A. "Points to Consider - Adolescents and HIV: Legal and Ethical Issues." Prepared for the Public Health Service Panel on Women, Adolescents, and Children with HIV Infection and AIDS. January 1992; OTA. June 1991. op cit.; DHHS. August 1991. op cit.

27 OTA. June 1991. op cit.

28 OTA. June 1991. op cit.

29 "Pennsylvania EPSDT Suit Filed." Health Advocate. Newsletter of the National Health Law Program. Los Angeles, CA. No. 170. Fall 1991; OTA. June 1991. op cit.

30 DHHS. August 1991. op cit.; English, A. 1992. op cit.

31 DHHS. August 1991. op cit.

32 English, A. 1992. op cit.

33 OTA. June 1991. op cit.

34 Public Law 101-508, The Omnibus Budget Reconciliation Act of 1990. Sec. 4601.

35 Public Law 101-508. op cit.

36 OTA. June 1991. op cit.

37 OTA. June 1991. op cit.

38 OTA. June 1991. op cit.

39 OTA. June 1991. op cit.

40 DHHS. National Center for Health Statistics. "Characteristics of Persons With and Without Health Care Coverage: United States, 1989." Advance Data No. 201. June 18, 1991.

41 AMA. 1991. op cit.

42 AMA. 1991. op cit.

43 OTA. Adolescent Health - Volume I: Summary and Policy Options. Washington, D.C.: U.S. Government Printing Office. April 1991.

44 OTA. April 1991. op cit.

45 OTA. June 1991. op cit.

46 OTA. June 1991. op cit.

47 OTA. June 1991. op cit.

48 OTA. June 1991. op cit.

49 Hein, K. Montefiore Medical Center. Personal Communication. March 16, 1992.

50 Cavanaugh, D. National Association of Community Health Centers. Personal Communication. March 20, 1992.

51 Cavanaugh, D. National Association of Community Health Centers. Personal Communication. March 27, 1992.

52 Kaiser, L. The Alan Guttmacher Institute. Personal Communication. March 20, 1992.

53 Kaiser, L. March 1992. op cit.

54 Kaiser, L. March 1992. op cit.

55 Sugarman, J. Center on Effective Services for Children. "Appropriations for Children's Programs, 1980, 1991 and 1992 -- Inflation Adjusted." Personal Communication. December 1991.

56 Gostin, L.O. "The AIDS Litigation Project. A National Review of Court and Human Rights Commission Decisions, Part I: The Social Impact of AIDS." Journal of the American Medical Association. Vol 263. No. 14. April 11, 1990.

57 Gostin, L.O. 1990. op cit.

58 Hein, K. "Fighting AIDS in Adolescents." Issues in Science and Technology, Spring 1991; Congress of the United States, Office of Technology Assessment. OTA. June 1991. op cit.

59 English, A. "Adolescents and HIV: Legal and Ethical Issues." National Center for Youth Law. San Francisco, CA. Prepared for the Public Health Service Panel on Women, Adolescents, and Children with HIV Infection and AIDS and the Working Group on Legal and Ethical Issues Related to HIV of the Public Health Service Task Force. January 1992; Henggeler, S.M., et al. Pediatric and Adolescent AIDS: Research Findings from the Social Sciences. Newbury Park, California: Sage. (in press).

60 Hein, K. Testimony at Hearing, AIDS and Teenagers: Emerging Issues. Select Committee on Children, Youth, and Families, U.S. House of Representatives, Washington, D.C. June 18, 1987.

61 English, A. "Adolescents and AIDS: Legal and Ethical Questions Multiply." Youth Law News. Vol. VIII, No. 6. November-December, 1987.

62 English, A. "Ethical/Legal Aspects of AIDS and STDs in Adolescents." Gallagher Lecture. Society for Adolescent Medicine. March 21, 1987.

63 English, A. 1992. op cit.

64 OTA. Adolescent Health - Vol. II: Crosscutting Issues in the Delivery of Health and Related Services. Washington, D.C.: U.S. Government Printing Office. November 1991; Hein, K. 1991. op cit.; English, A. 1992. op cit.; Garrison, J. "Services and Treatment Issues *Recommendations of the Work Group.*" Journal of Adolescent Health Care. Vol. 10. No. 3. Supplement 1989.

65 Rotheram-Borus, M.J. Testimony at Hearing, The Risky Business of Adolescence: How to Help Teens Stay Safe. Select Committee on Children, Youth, and Families. U.S. House of Representatives. Washington, D.C. June 17, 1991.

66 English, A. January 1992. op cit.

67 North, R. "Legal Authority for HIV Testing of Adolescents." Journal of Adolescent Health Care. Vol 11. No. 2. Gittler, J. et al. "Adolescent Health Care Decision-Making: The Law and Public Police." Washington, D.C.: Carnegie Council on Adolescent Development. 1990. (Cited by English, A. 1992. op cit.)

68 English, A. 1992. op cit.

69 North, R. 1990. op cit.

70 English, A. 1992. op cit.

71 English, A. 1992. op cit.

72 English, A. 1992. op cit.; North, R.L. 1990. op. cit.; Gittler, J., et al. 1990. op cit.

73 Melton, G. "Ethical and Legal Issues in Research and Intervention." Journal of Adolescent Health Care. Vol. 10. No. 3. 1989.

74 Melton, G. 1989. op cit.

75 English, A. 1992. op cit.

76 Shafer, M.A. Testimony at Hearing, AIDS and Teenagers: Emerging Issues. Select Committee on Children, Youth, and Families. U.S. House of Representatives. Washington, D.C. June 18, 1987; Hein, K. June 1987. op cit.

77 Hein, K. "Mandatory HIV Testing of Youth -- A Lose-Lose Proposition." Journal of the American Medical Association. Vol. 266. No. 17. November 6, 1991.

78 Shafer, M. 1987. op cit.

79 Hein, K. November 1991. op cit.

80 Mark, V. Testimony at Hearing, AIDS and Teenagers: Emerging Issues. Select Committee on Children, Youth, and Families. U.S. House of Representatives. Washington, D.C. June 18, 1987.

81 English, A. Personal Communication. March 1992; Hein, K. 1987. op cit.; Hein, K. November 1991. op cit.; Rogers, D. and Osborn, J. "Another Approach to the AIDS Epidemic." New England Journal of Medicine. Vol. 321. 1991.

82 English, A. March 1992. op cit.

83 English, A. "AIDS Testing and Epidemiology for Youth-Recommendations of the Work Group." Journal of Adolescent Health Care. Vol. 10. No. 3. Supplement. May 1989.

84 Massachusetts Department of Public Health. Comprehensive Guidelines Adolescent HIV Antibody Counseling and Testing. Draft July 1990; Rosenfeld, S. Personal Communication. June 1991.

85 CDC. "Education and Foster Care of Children Infected With Human T-Lymphotropic Virus Type III/Lymphadenopathy-Associated Virus." Morbidity and Mortality Weekly Report. Vol. 34. No. 34. August 30, 1985; American Academy of Pediatrics,

Committee on Infectious Diseases. "Health Guidelines for the Attendance in Day Care and Foster Care Settings of Children Infected with Human Immunodeficiency Virus." Pediatrics. Vol. 79. No. 3. March 1987.

86 CDC. August 1985. op cit.

87 AAP. Committee on Infectious Diseases. March 1987. op cit.

88 English, A. 1987(b). op cit.

89 CDC. August 1985. op cit.

90 CDC. August 1985. op cit.

91 National Association of State Boards of Education. "NASBE Releases AIDS Survey." June 1987.

92 CDC. August 1985. op cit.

Appendix A

GLOSSARY OF ABBREVIATIONS AND TERMS[(a)]

I. Abbreviations:

ADAMHA	Alcohol, Drug Abuse, and Mental Health Administration (PHS)
AFL	Adolescent Family Life (program under Title XX of the Public Health Service Act)
AHCPR	Agency for Health Care Policy Research (DHHS)
AIDS	acquired immunodeficiency syndrome
BHCDA	Bureau of Health Care Delivery and Assistance (HRSA)
BHPr	Bureau of Health Professionals (HRSA)
BHRD	Bureau of Health Resource Development (HRSA)
BIA	Bureau of Indian Affairs (U.S. Department of the Interior)
BMCH	Bureau of Maternal and Child Health (HRSA)
CASSP	Child and Adolescent Service System Program (NIMH)
CDC	Centers for Disease Control (PHS)
CHC	community health center
CRS	Congressional Research Service (Library of Congress)

(a) The abbreviations and terms included in this glossary were developed by the Office of Technology Assessment for its Adolescent Health report. A few additional abbreviations have been added to clarify terms used by this report. Used with permission.

DAWN	Drug Abuse Warning Network (NIDA)
DHHS	U.S. Department of Health and Human Services
DMCH	Department of Maternal and Child Health
EPSDT	Early and Periodic Screening, Diagnosis, and Treatment program (Medicaid)
GAO	General Accounting Office (U.S. Congress)
HCFA	Health Care Financing Administration (DHHS)
HIV	human immunodeficiency virus (AIDS virus)
HRSA	Health Resources and Services Administration (PHS)
IHS	Indian Health Service
IOM	Institute of Medicine (NAS)
IV	intravenous
NAIEP	National AIDS Information and Education Program (CDC)
NAPO	National AIDS Program Office (DHHS)
NAS	National Academy of Sciences
NCHS	National Center for Health Statistics (CDC)
NCCDPHP	National Center for Chronic Disease Prevention and Health Promotion (CDC)
NCI	National Cancer Institute (NIH)
NCID	National Center for Infectious Diseases (NIH)
NCNR	National Center for Nursing Research (NIH)
NCRR	National Center for Research Resources (NIH)
NCPS	National Center for Prevention Services (CDC)

NDATUS	National Drug and Alcoholism Treatment Unit Survey (ADAMHA)
NHIS	National Health Interview Survey (NCHS)
NIAAA	National Institute on Alcohol Abuse and Alcoholism (ADAMHA)
NIAID	National Institute of Allergy and Infectious Diseases (NIH)
NICHD	National Institute of Child Health and Human Development (NIH)
NIDA	National Institute on Drug Abuse (ADAMHA)
NIDR	National Institute on Dental Research (NIH)
NIH	National Institutes of Health (PHS)
NIMH	National Institute of Mental Health (ADAMHA)
NSAM	National Survey of Adolescent Males
NSFG	National Survey of Family Growth (NCHS)
OAP	Office of Adolescent Pregnancy (DHHS)
ODPHP	Office of Disease Prevention and Health Promotion (DHHS)
OJJDP	Office of Juvenile Justice and Delinquency Prevention (U.S. Department of Justice)
OSAP	Office for Substance Abuse Prevention (ADAMHA)
OTA	Office of Technology Assessment (U.S. Congress)
PHS	Public Health Service (DHHS)
PID	pelvic inflammatory disease
SPRANS	special projects of regional and national significance (under Title V of the Social Security Act)

STD sexually transmitted disease

YRBSS Youth Risk Behavioral Surveillance System (CDC)

II. Terms:

Abstinence from sexual activity: Refraining from sexual intercourse, one approach to the prevention of sexually transmitted disease (STD), AIDS, and pregnancy.

Access: Potential and actual entry of a population into the health care delivery system.

Adolescence: Definitions of adolescence vary, and many observers agree that a definition based on age alone is not sufficient. Adolescence typically takes place during the second decade of life, and is initiated by puberty, although physical and other changes occur (i.e, in height, weight, head size, facial structure, facial expression, and cognitive abilities). As used in this report, adolescence most often refers to the period of life from ages 10 through 18.

African-American: See Black.

AIDS (acquired immunodeficiency syndrome): A disease characterized by a deficiency of the immune system caused by human immunodeficiency virus (HIV). The primary defect in AIDS is an acquired, persistent, quantitative functional depression within the T4 subset of lymphocytes. This depression often leads to infections caused by micro-organisms that usually do not produce infections in individuals with normal immunity. HIV infection can be transmitted from one infected individual to another by means that include the sharing of a contaminated intravenous needle and engaging in unprotected sexual intercourse (i.e., intercourse without the use of condoms) with an infected person.

Alcohol, Drug Abuse, and Mental Health (ADM) Block Grant Program: The major Federal program providing funds to States for outpatient alcohol, drug abuse, and mental health treatment programs. (Funds are not allowed to be used for inpatient services.) States receive a share of the ADM block grant appropriation through a formula based in part on the size of the State population (Subpart 1, part B of Title XIX of the Public Health Service Act). The ADM Block Grant Program is administered by the Office of Treatment Improvement in the Alcohol, Drug Abuse, and Mental Health Administration in DHHS.

American Indian or Alaska Native: A person having origins in any of the original peoples of North American and maintaining cultural identification through tribal affiliation or community recognition.

Appropriation (by Congress): An Act of Congress that authorizes one or more Federal agencies to incur obligations and make payments from the general fund or various special funds of the U.S. Treasury. Appropriations do not represent funds available in the Treasury but are limitations on the amounts that agencies may obligate during the time period set in the law.

Asian or Pacific Islander: A person having origins in any of the original peoples of the Far East, Southeast Asia, the Indian subcontinent, or the Pacific Islands. The area includes China, India, Japan, Korea, the Philippine Island, and Samoa.

Authorization (by Congress): Substantive legislation that creates or continues a Federal agency or program for an indefinite or specified period of time. It may prescribe funding methods, allow a particular type of expenditure, or limit the level of budget authority.

AZT: See zidovudine.

Black: A person having origins in any of the Black racial groups in Africa. Normally excludes persons of Hispanic origin except for tabulations produced by the Bureau of the Census, which are noted accordingly.

Block grants: Sums of Federal funds allotted to State agencies (e.g., education, health) which may be passed on to local agencies. States determine the mix of services provided and the population served and are accountable to the Federal Government only to the extent that funds are spent in accordance with program requirements. Sometimes, however, set-asides are required for specific population groups.

Child and Adolescent Service System Program (CASSP): A small program, administered by the National Institute of Mental Health in DHHS, that was created by Congress in 1984 to promote greater coordination among public and private agencies providing services to children and adolescents with mental health problems.

Chlamydia infection: Any sexually transmitted disease (STD) that is characterized by infection with the bacterial agent Chlamydia trachomatous. Such infection, which may be asymptomatic or accompanied by symptoms such as dysuria (difficult urination), penile or vaginal discharge, and urinary frequency, can potentially lead to complications that include urethral stricture, urethritis, salpingitis, epididymitis, infertility, and adverse obstetrical outcomes. Methods of prevention include the avoidance of multiple sexual partners. Treatment is with antibiotics. Chlamydia is the most common type of sexually transmitted disease among U.S. adolescents.

Cocaine: A psychoactive substance derived from coca leaves. Several types of coca preparations are used for their psychoactive properties: coca leaves (chewed), coca paste (smoked), cocaine hydrochloride powder (inhaled or injected), and cocaine alkaloid-"freebase" or "crack" (smoked).

Cognitive-behavioral skills training program: Prevention and/or health promotion interventions that are based on the idea that problem behavior and emotional distress sometimes result from an ability to develop and maintain positive social relationships due to deficits in social skills. Interpersonal cognitive problem solving programs focus on processes such as interpreting social cues and others' intentions, generating alternative solutions, and means-ends thinking. Behavioral social skills training interventions focus on teaching specific behaviors such as entering a peer group, accepting criticism, giving compliments and resisting peer pressure. Many programs incorporate aspects of both types of training, often as a part of a school curriculum and done in small groups of students.

Community health center (CHC): An organization that provides primary health care and other health-related services to individuals in the local community. As of 1989, there were about 1,200 community health centers providing services at more than 2,000 sites throughout the country. Roughly half of these centers were receiving Federal grants under Section 330 of the Public Health Service Act, which authorizes grants to public and private nonprofit organizations that provide primary health care to populations or areas that are "medically undeserved."

Comparison group: In evaluation research, a group that does not receive the "experimental" intervention or program, but receives no or a different intervention.

Comprehensive services for adolescents: The elements of comprehensive health and related services for adolescents are not entirely agreed upon. They include, at a minimum, care for acute physical illnesses, general medical examinations in preparation for involvement in athletics, mental health counseling, laboratory tests, reproductive health care, family counseling, prescriptions, advocacy, and coordination of care; the more comprehensive may include educational services, vocational services, legal assistance, recreational opportunities, and child care services and parenting education for adolescent parents.

Condom: A sheath commonly made of rubber worn over the penis for the purpose of preventing pregnancy or preventing the transmission of human immunodeficiency virus (HIV) or particular types of sexually transmitted diseases (STDs).

Contraceptives or contraceptive methods: Methods of preventing pregnancy other than abstinence from sexual activity. Such methods include periodic abstinence (rhythm method); control of ejaculation (coitus interruptus); the use of spermicidal chemicals in jellies or creams; mechanical barriers (e.g., condoms, caps, or diaphragms); prevention of implantation (e.g., intrauterine device); the use of synthetic hormones to control the female reproductive cycle; and sterilization of the male or female partner. Various methods vary in terms of their effectiveness in preventing pregnancy, their side effects, and their noncontraceptive benefits such as protection from sexually transmitted diseases (STDs).

Decisionmaking skills: Skills relevant to the ability to make rational, health-promoting decisions about one's life. Often a part of life skills training interventions.

Delinquent acts by adolescents: Two broad categories of acts committed by adolescents: 1) acts that would be considered crimes if committed by an adult (ranging from minor offenses such as disorderly conduct to serious offenses such as aggravated assault); and 2) status offenses, which are considered offenses only when committed by minors (e.g., running away from home, truancy).

Demographic factors: Age, gender, race, ethnicity, geographic location and socioeconomic status are typically defined as demographic factors.

Detoxification: The recovery, or the process of bringing about the recovery, of a patient from a state of dependence on alcohol or other drug. **Medical detoxification** is the use of medication under the supervision of medical personnel to systematically reduce or eliminate the effects of alcohol in the body in a hospital or other 24-hour facility. **Social detoxification** is to systematically reduce or eliminate the effects of alcohol in the body on a drug-free basis, in a specialized nonmedical facility by trained medical personnel with physician services available when required. **Drug detoxification** is the period of planned withdrawal from drug dependency supported by the use of a prescribed medication (e.g., methadone).

Developmentally appropriate: Health promotion, prevention, and treatment services and environments designed so that they fit the emotional, behavioral/experiential, and intellectual levels of the individual who is to benefit from the service. Because of the asynchronous development within even individual adolescents (as well as individuals in other age categories), designing programs so that they are developmentally appropriate is a distinct challenge.

Diaphragm: A prescription contraceptive method that involves the insertion of a dome-shaped rubber cap with a flexible rim into the vagina prior to intercourse. Spermicidal cream or jelly is placed in the dome before insertion. The diaphragm and spermicide combination probably provides some protection against sexually transmitted disease (STD), including pelvic inflammatory disease (PID).

Drug Abuse Warning Network (DAWN): A system that collects data on emergency room visits and deaths related to drug use from a sample of hospital emergency rooms and medical examiner facilities that report data for each "drug abuse" patient or death encountered by medical examiners. The DAWN system is designed primarily as an early warning system to monitor drug abuse patterns and health hazards associated with drug use and to detect new abuse entities and new combinations. The system is maintained by the National Institute on Drug Abuse in DHHS.

Ethnicity: A term used to indicate national origin (e.g., Hispanic, Asian). Most ethnic-specific census and health status information in available only for individuals of Hispanic origin.

Family life education: Ideally, a curriculum, program, or framework for helping young people make responsible choices and decisions by providing accurate and age-appropriate information about human sexuality, and by exploring the attitudes, behaviors, and value systems that shape the development of healthy sexuality. May include teaching of skills in communication, responsible decisionmaking, and assertiveness. See life skills training. Family life education is the more current and encompassing term for programs formerly, and now sometimes, known as sex education.

Family planning programs authorized by Title X of the Public Health Service Act: Title X, established by the Family Planning Services and Population Research Act of 1970, funds public or private nonprofit entities that operate voluntary family planning projects; funds training for personnel to improve the delivery of family planning services; promotes service delivery improvement through research; and develops and disseminates information on family planning. Contraceptives may be distributed without parental consent or notification, but the use of Title X funds for abortion as a method of family planning has been prohibited by statute and regulations. Low-income individuals are targeted as a priority group for receiving services. Although projects funded by Title X do not focus a broad range of family planning services to all who want them, including adolescents.

Family planning services: A range of services intended to help individuals plan when to have children, which typically include birth control information and counseling, provision of contraceptives, pregnancy testing and counseling, gynecological examinations, and referrals for related services. Such services are available through a variety of public and health providers that include Title X planning clinics as well as more general health services settings.

Federally funded runaway and homeless youth centers: Locally controlled facilities that receive Federal funds under the Federal Runaway and Homeless Youth Act (Title III of the Juvenile Justice and Delinquency Prevention Act) administered by the Administration for Children, Youth, and Families within the Office of Human Development Services of DHHS as well as other funds. In fiscal year 1987, there were 307 federally funded runaway and homeless youth centers throughout the country. Federally funded runaway and homeless youth centers provide emergency shelter (for up to 15 days), counseling, and other services to runaway or otherwise homeless youth.

Federal poverty level: The official U.S. Government definition of poverty based on cash income levels for families of different sizes. Responsibility for changing poverty concepts and definitions rests with the Office of Management and Budget.

Financial access (to health services): In this Report, used to refer to aspects of access that have to do with health insurance coverage and ability to pay for services.

Foster care: In its broadest sense, the placement of children in foster family homes, group homes, group child care facilities and residential treatment centers by the child welfare system. Most children in foster care are placed in foster family homes, that is, with a foster parent or parents and the parents' own or other foster children. Children and adolescents placed in foster care have been removed from their homes because of abuse, neglect, or abandonment, and they have either been adjudicated "dependent" by the counts or voluntarily placed in foster care by their families.

Gonorrhea: A sexually transmitted disease (STD) characterized by infection with the bacterial agent Neisseria gonorrhea. Gonorrhea, which may be asymptomatic or accompanied by vaginal/penile discharge, abdominal pain, or other symptoms, can potentially lead to complications that include disseminated gonococcal infection(e.g., septicemia), pelvic inflammatory disease (PID), epididymitis, and infertility or sterility. Spermicides and condoms offer some protection from this disease. Treatment is with antibiotics. Gonorrhea is the second most common type of sexually transmitted disease among U.S. adolescents.

Hispanic: A person who identifies himself or herself as of Hispanic origin, or, less typically, individuals with Hispanic surnames identified by others (e.g., health care providers identifying patients in surveys) as being of Hispanic origin. Hispanics can be individuals whose families or ancestors have emigrated directly from Mexico, Puerto Rico, Cuba, Central or South America, Spain, or other Spanish culture or origin, regardless of race.

Homelessness: The state of being without one's own home, either on one's own, with one's family, living on the street or in a shelter or other temporary situation (e.g., with relatives or friends).

Human immunodeficiency virus (HIV): The virus that causes AIDS. Two distinct subtypes of HIV have been identified: HIV-1 was first isolated in 1983 and has a worldwide distribution. HIV-2 was first isolated in 1986 and is found mainly in West Africa.

Iatrogenic effects: Adverse conditions that are induced inadvertently by a health care provider or by the treatment.

Illicit drugs: In this report, unless otherwise noted, a term used to refer to drugs which are not legally available to adults (e.g., marijuana, cocaine, hallucinogens, PCP, heroin) or the illicit use of prescription drugs to get high or for other mental effects. The NIDA Household

Survey on Drug Abuse defines illicit drugs as "marijuana, cocaine, inhalants, hallucinogens, PCP, heroin, or nonmedical use of psychotherapeutics." The Monitoring the Future/High School Seniors Survey defines illicit drugs as "marijuana, cocaine, heroin, or any use which is not under a doctor's orders of other opiates, stimulants, or tranquilizers."

Incidence: In health epidemiology, the measure of the number of new cases of a particular disease or condition occurring in a population during a given period of time. Incidence rate is the number of new cases of specified disease divided by the number of people in a population over a specified period of time, usually 1 year.

Indians: American Indians in the continental United States, and American Indians, Aleuts and Eskimos in Alaska.

Intravenous drug use: The intake of drugs (e.g. heroin, cocaine, amphetamines) directly into the veins, usually by means of a needle injection.

Job Corps: A program administered by the Employment and Training Administration in the U.S. Department of Labor, providing employment and training in primarily residential centers for socioeconomically disadvantaged young people ages 12 to 21.

Juvenile: A young person who has not yet reached the age at which he or she should be treated as an adult for purposes of criminal law. In some States, this age is 17. In law, the terms juvenile and minor are usually used in different contexts (juvenile when referring to young legal offenders and minor when referring to legal majority or capacity).

Juvenile justice facilities: Custodial facilities for juveniles. These can be classified along several, often overlapping, dimensions that include purpose, term of stay, type of environment (institutional or open), and sponsorship (public or private). **Juvenile detention facilities and shelters** typically hold adolescents while they are awaiting adjudication or after adjudication placement. **Juvenile correctional facilities** hold adolescents after adjudication for the purpose of commitment or for supervision and treatment. **Short-term juvenile facilities,** which include juvenile detention facilities and shelters, are typically used for adolescents who are awaiting adjudication, adolescents who have been sentenced to short period of confinement, or adolescents who are awaiting transfer to long-term placements. **Long-term facilities,** which range from training schools to less restrictive facilities such as ranches, forestry camps, or farms to even less restrictive halfway houses and group homes, primarily serve adolescents who have been adjudicated. **Public juvenile facilities** are under the direct administration and operational control of State or local government and staffed by governmental employees. **Private juvenile facilities** are either profitmaking or nonprofit and subject to governmental licensing but are under the direct administration and operational control of private enterprise; such facilities may receive substantial public funding in addition to their support from private sources.

Juvenile offender: A juvenile who has violated the law.

Latino: Of Latin American origin.

Legal access (to health services): In this report, used to refer to aspects of access that have to do with consent and confidentiality.

Life skills training: The formal teaching of the requisite skills for surviving, living with others, and succeeding in a complex society. Life skills training interventions emphasize the teaching of social competence, cognitive skills, and decisionmaking skills.

Longitudinal studies: Studies that examine the development of individuals or families or groups over a period of time.

Maternal and Child Health (MCH) Services Block Grant Program: A Federal block grant program authorized under Title V of the Social Security Act, that supports the provision of health services to mothers and children, especially those with low income or living in areas with limited availability of health services. Funds are provided to States, which in turn may provide them to local health departments. Created by the Omnibus Budget Reconciliation Act of 1981, the MCH Block Grant consolidated several categorical grant programs into one block grant. The MCH Block Grant is administered at the Federal level by the Bureau of Maternal and Child Health in the Health Resources and Services Administration in DHHS.

Medicaid: A federally aided, State-administered program, authorized under Title XIX of the Social Security Act, that provides medical assistance for low-income people meeting specific income and family structure requirements. Medicaid covers and estimated 4.5 million individuals ages 10 to 18 and is the major health care financing mechanism for the adolescents in low-income families.

Mentoring: The practice of acting over time as a guide, tutor or coach, and sometimes as an advocate for another, typically not biologically related, person.

Metropolitan Statistical Area: As defined by the U.S. Office of Management and Budget, a county or group of counties that includes either a city of at least 50,000 residents, or an urbanized area with at least 50,000 people that itself is part of a county/counties with at least 100,000 total residents.

Mortality rate: A measure derived by dividing the number of deaths in a population in a given period by the resident population at the middle of that period. It is expressed as the number of deaths per 1,000 population. The rate may be restricted to deaths in specific age, race, sex, or geographic groups (e.g., 15 deaths per 1,000 persons ages 15 to 19), or it may be related to the entire population.

National Survey of Family Growth (NSFG): A household interview survey that has collected data from U.S. women of childbearing age (ages 15 through 44) in four cycles since 1974. NSFG collects data on the demographic and social factors associated with childbearing, adoption, and maternal and child health-including sexual activity, contraception and sterilization, marriage, pregnancy loss, and use of medical care for family planning and prenatal care. NSFG is conducted by the National Center for Health Statistics in DHHS.

NIDA Household Survey on Drug Abuse: A household survey, sponsored since 1974 by the National Institute of Drug Abuse within DHHS, that collect data on the in use of marijuana and other illicit drugs, tobacco, and alcohol among the U.S. population 12 years of age and over living in households in the coterminous United States. Youths (12 to 17 years of age) and young adults (ages 18 to 25 years of age) are oversampled, as are Blacks and Hispanics.

Outcome evaluation: Measures an intervention's result (e.g., increased knowledge, changed behavior).

Parental consent requirement: As used in this report, a legal requirement, grounded in common law, that a parent or other guardian of a minor child must give prior to consent to the delivery of medical or surgical care to that child.

Peer tutoring: Using older or same age students to work individually with students to teach a particular content area.

Pelvic inflammatory disease (PID) A sexually transmitted disease (STD) among females, the symptoms of which include abdominal pain, fever, chills, vomiting, foul-smelling discharge, and postcoital bleeding. Potential complications include sterility, chronic pain, chronic infections, and even death. Methods of prevention include limiting the number of sexual partners, using of condoms, and avoiding the use of intrauterine contraceptive devices. Treatment is with antibiotics.

Physical abuse: Physical violence, including kicking, biting, hitting with one's fist, beating, burning, or scalding, and using a weapon.

Physical neglect: As defined by DHHS's National Center on Child Abuse and Neglect, physical neglect can take seven forms: refusal to provide health care for physical problems, as recommended by a competent health care professional; delay in providing health care for a serious physical problem; desertion of a child without arranging for reasonable care and supervision (abandonment); other blatant refusals of custody, such as permanent or indefinite expulsion of a child from the home; other custody issues, such as chronically and repeatedly leaving a child with others for days or weeks at a time; inadequate supervision; and other physical neglect, such as conspicuous inattention to avoidable hazards in the home.

Prevalence: In health epidemiology, a measure of the number of individuals in a given population who have a specific disease or other condition at a designated time (or during a particular period).

Preventive health services: Services intended to prevent the occurrence of a problem (e.g., disease or condition). Preventive services typically recommended for adolescents include routine physical examinations, immunizations, and certain diagnostic tests (e.g., hematocrit, urinalysis), and preventive procedures including pap smears and screening for sexually transmitted diseases among the sexually active.

Primary care: Optimally, primary care includes the following elements: first contact care, comprehensive care, coordinated or integrated care, and care that is longitudinal over time rather than episodic. First contact care is the extent to which a patient contracts the source of care whenever he or she perceived a new need for care. Coordination of care entails a health care provider's ability to provide for continuity of information from visits to other providers (e.g., specialists and emergency facilities) as well as from earlier visits to him or herself. Longitudinality of care is the extent to which a provider serves as a source of care over time regardless of the presence or absence of a particular type of problem.

Process evaluation: The [documentation] aspects of a program's implementation and operation.

Puberty: The period of becoming first capable of reproducing sexually, marked by maturing of the genital organs, development of secondary sex characteristics (e.g., breasts, pubic hair), and in humans and higher primates, the first occurrence of menstruation in the female.

Race: Races can be distinguished by usually inherited physical and physiological characteristics without regard to language or culture. Beginning in 1976, the Federal Government's data systems classified individuals into the following racial groups: White, Black, Asian or Pacific Islander, or American Indian and Alaska Native.

Racial and ethnic minorities: In this report, individuals who are not "White, non-Hispanic." Includes African American, Asian, Hispanic, and Alaska Native individuals.

Reproductive health care: Can include a wide range of services related to the male or female reproductive systems, including gynecological treatment services (i.e., examination and treatment of the female reproductive organs), and preventive services related to the use of contraception (e.g., counseling, prescribing contraceptive methods, dispensing contraceptives).

Risk-taking behavior: An activity that may involve a risk to one's health. For adolescents especially, risk-taking generally carries a negative connotation, but some risk taking is essential to the further development of competence, and thus some risk-taking can have positive health and other benefits.

Runaway: A young person who is away from home at least overnight without the permission of a parent or caretaker.

Safer sex practices: Sexual practices designed to avoid actual and potential transmission of HIV infection and other sexually transmitted diseases (e.g., avoiding exchange of body fluids, use of condoms).

School-linked health center (SLHC): Any school health center that provides a wide range of medical and counseling services for students (and sometimes for the family members of students and/or school drop-outs) and is located either on or near school grounds and is associated with the school. Some SLHCs also provide a wider range of services (e.g., child care, employment training, tutoring, social services, recreational opportunities).

Seropositive: Showing a high level of antibody.

Seroprevalence: Prevalence based on blood tests.

Sex education: Instruction about human sexual development, the process of reproduction, and related topics. Currently, the content and process of many sex education programs have been broadened, and such programs are often known as family life education.

Sexual abuse: As defined by DHHS's National Center on Child Abuse and Neglect, sexual abuse can take three forms: actual penile penetration; molestation with genital contact; and other unspecified acts not known to have involved actual genital contact (e.g., fondling of breasts or buttocks, exposure), or inadequate or inappropriate supervision of a child's voluntary sexual activities.

Sexual activity rate: As typically used in the literature, the number of individuals who have ever had sexual intercourse, per some population base.

Sexually active: As typically used in the literature, sexually active denoted ever having had sexual intercourse (as opposed to currently being sexually active).

Sexually transmitted disease (STD): Any infections disease transmitted through sexual intercourse or genital contact. Examples are chlamydial infection, gonorrhea, herpes genitalis, pelvic inflammatory disease (PID), syphilis, and AIDS. Formerly (and sometimes, in law) called venereal disease.

Social services: Services provided in order to support the functioning of individuals or family units, including those services termed: 1) "supportive" or "protective services"; 2) supplementary (i.e. financial assistance, home aid services, respite care); and 3) "substitute" services (e.g., shelter services, foster care, adoption).

Social Support: Can involve the provision of any or all of 1) supportive aid, including practical services and material benefits; 2) personal affirmation, including feedback that raises self-esteem and strengthens personal identity; and 3) supportive affect, particularly affection, caring, and nurturance.

Socioeconomic status: Generally used in this report as a synonym for income levels, typically those of an adolescent's family of origin. In some cases, however, socioeconomic status refers more broadly to a combination of factors such as father's education, mother's education, family income, household items, etc.

Spermicides: Contraceptive agents that work by killing sperm. Spermicides come in various forms (e.g., jellies or creams to be used in diaphragms, contraceptive vaginal sponges, spermicidal condoms). Spermicides decrease the transmission of some sexually transmitted diseases (STDs), including gonorrhea.

Statistically significant: A judgement, based on commonly agreed to statistical principles, that there is relatively little likelihood (typically from below 1 to below 5 percent) that an observed relationship between or among variables has occurred by chance.

Street kid: A long-term runaway, thrownaway, or otherwise homeless child or adolescent who has become adept at fending for him or herself "on the street," usually by illegal activities.

Survival sex: Engaging in sexual intercourse in exchange for food, shelter, money, or drugs.

Syphilis: A sexually transmitted disease (STD) caused by the bacterial agent Treponema pallidum, resulting in symptoms including chancre (primary syphilis); skin rash, malaise, anorexia, nausea (secondary syphilis); and eventually, central nervous system abnormalities and other serious problems (tertiary syphilis).

Thrownaway: A child or adolescent who has been told to leave the household, has been abandoned or deserted, or who has run away and no effort has been made to recover him or her.

Title X family planning clinics: Family planning clinics that receive funds under Title X of the Public Health Service Act.

Title X program (Family Planning Services and Research Program) under the Public Health Services Act: A Federal program that provides Federal grants to help support about 4,000 family planning clinics operated by public or private nonprofit entities across the country, as well as funds for training and research to improve the delivery of family planning services. the Title X program is administered at the Federal level by the Office of Population Affairs within DHHS. Family planning clinics that receive Title X funds offer contraceptives and other family planning services (not including abortion). The services offered by family planning clinics are provided free or at rates determined on a sliding-fee scale and are confidential.

About one-third of the patients of such clinics are adolescents ages 15 to 19.

Title XX program (Adolescent Family Life Program) under the Public Health Service Act: A Federal program that awards Federal grants for demonstration projects that seek to prevent adolescent pregnancy by encouraging adolescents, within the context of the family, to abstain from premarital sexual activity and for demonstration projects that provide health and social services for pregnant or patenting adolescents. The Title XX program is administered by the Office of Population Affairs with DHHS.

Treatment services: Services intended to cure or ameliorate the effects of a disease or other health problem once the problem has occurred.

Unprotected sexual intercourse: Sexual intercourse without precautions taken to prevent pregnancy or the transmission of AIDS or other sexually transmitted diseases.

Youth Risk Behavior Surveillance System (YRBSS): This system, recently developed by the Centers for Disease Control in DHHS, will monitor the prevalence of priority risk behaviors among samples of school-aged adolescents by collecting data from a periodic school-based survey combined with special supplemental data on youth risk behavior from the National Health Interview Survey conducted by DHHS. The system will be implemented in 1991, 1995, and 2000.

Zidovudine (Retrovir^{R}): A drug used to reduce symptoms prolonging the lives of person infected with human immunodeficiency virus (HIV). This drug was formerly called idothymidine (AZT).

SUBJECT INDEX